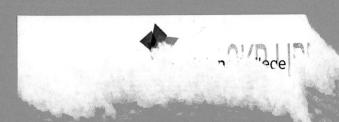

10-MINUTE
HAIRSTYLES

50 step-by-step looks

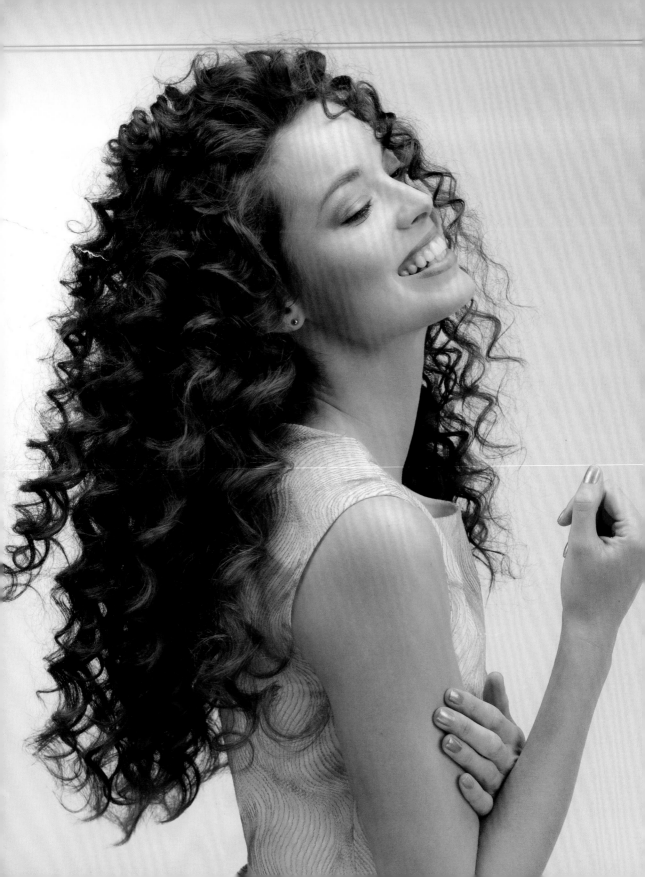

André Märtens

10-MINUTE
HAIRSTYLES

50 step-by-step looks

With photos by Eugen Mai

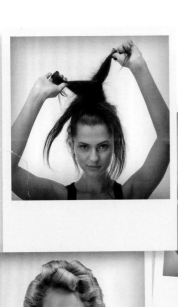

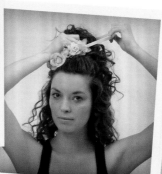

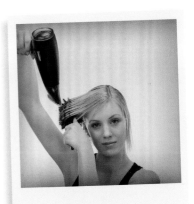

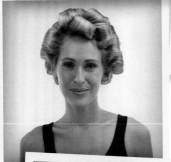

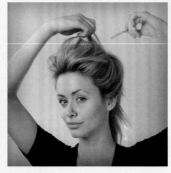

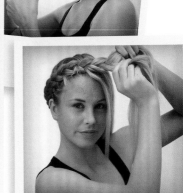

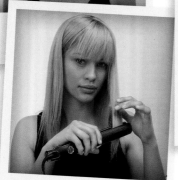

CONTENTS

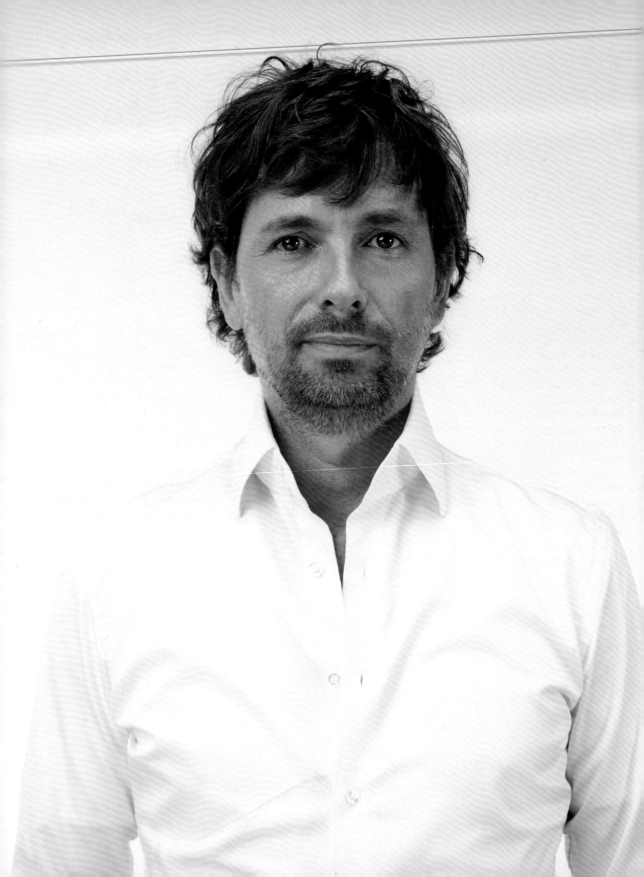

FOREWORD

When I was doing my training, you didn't go "to the hairdresser", you went "for a perm". Now almost a no-go style, it shows just how much tastes and fashion are always changing. Nowadays, hair is supposed to look as natural as possible: we respect and build on the structure that's already there and, as well as keeping up with the current trends, we want a look that's right for us. But, hand on heart, how often have you gone in search of the ideal haircut or the perfect style for your type? Painstakingly growing your hair long, only for split and thinning ends to make you get rid of it again – usually following a moment of realization: "I can't stand this scraggly mess – I have to get to the hairdresser's right now!" Or have you spontaneously decided to dye your brunette hair strawberry blonde, because it was the celebrity "in" colour – only to realize that the shade was really unflattering against your rosy complexion?

My advice? Big changes aren't the only things that can liven up a look. If you've found a good basic cut and a good length for everyday styling, there are countless ways to reinvent yourself and your whole appearance on a daily basis. That might mean a different parting or a soft colour kick, a trendy chignon, sophisticated braid, or putting gentle temporary waves in naturally sleek hair.

In my years of working on Berlin Fashion Week, I've seen a lot of current trends, and have often been called upon to transform hairstyles in very little time. Inspired by this, on the following pages I will show you the best styles for hair of every length, type, and structure – from business chic to a glamorous evening updo – all easy to manage in ten minutes, thanks to the clear, step-by-step instructions. The brush symbols tell you how difficult each style is. One brush means "very easy; suitable for complete beginners"; two brushes mean "intermediate – some experience required", and three brushes denotes a more challenging style – although even these are easy to master with a little practice.

Have fun trying out the styles, being brave, and reinventing yourself!

Yours,

HAIR CARE

The be-all and end-all for beautiful hair is finding the right care products. Shampoo, conditioner, and hair masks are little miracle-workers. They can smooth frizz, temporarily patch together split ends, or sooth an irritated scalp. They volumize fine hair, and give stressed-out manes their shine back.

SHAMPOO

The main ingredients of shampoos are salt, water, perfumes, and detergents, which are also called tensides. These days, tensides are so mild that you can wash your hair every day. In choosing the right shampoo, you should consider the needs of your scalp. Does it tend to be oily, dry, or flaky? Structural problems with your hair, such as split or dry ends, brittle hair, or frizz, on the other hand, are a job for conditioner, or an occasional nourishing hair masque. Important: wet hair thoroughly before shampooing. Work a blob of shampoo and a little water into a lather between your hands, and gently massage it into your scalp. The shampoo running down your hair as you rinse will be enough to clean the ends. Always rinse out shampoo very thoroughly, particularly from your roots. Residue can make hair look dull or even give you an itchy scalp. There's a shampoo out there for every hair type – and if in doubt, ask the experts.

PEELING SHAMPOO

Peeling shampoos are a kind of deep cleanse for your hair. They contain micro beads, strong tensides, or fruit acids, which free your hair and scalp from build-ups of styling products and silicon. They can even remove excess pigments if a home hair dye has come out too dark or too red. However, peeling shampoos don't really nourish your hair, and can easily dry it out, so they should only be used occasionally.

TWO-IN-ONE SHAMPOO

Two-in-one shampoos are a relic from the 1980s, combining shampoo and conditioner. The problem with them used to be that they often contained insoluble silicon, which built up every time you washed your hair. After a while, it made hair limp, heavy, and straggly. Today, they usually contain soluble silicone, which can be washed out. My tip is to check out the "INCI" list of ingredients. Insoluble silicones include dimethicone, cyclomethicone, cyclopentoxilase, and dimothiconol. The soluble (ie unproblematic) silicones include amodimethicone, polysiloxane, PEG/PPG-14/4 dimethicone and dimethicone copolyol.

DRY SHAMPOO

This miracle product from the 1970s is currently making a big comeback. Dry shampoos are usually available as sprays, containing rice starch and silicon. The starch absorbs excess oil from your scalp, making hair look fresh even a day after washing. One bonus side-effect of dry shampoos is that they give your hair volume and manageability. Important: use dry shampoo sparingly, concentrating on your roots. Massage it in with your fingers and brush out thoroughly. If any residue is left in your hair, it can give it an unwanted matte finish, or make it look like it's covered in a grey film.

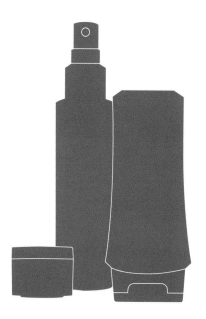

CONDITIONER

Conditioners should optimize the condition of your hair. They work on the surface of your hair, smoothing the outer layer to make it sleeker, shinier, and easier to comb. Conditioner should be used straight after washing, on damp hair. Apply it to the body and ends of your hair, but never to the roots. Most conditioners are formulated so that one to three minutes on your hair is sufficient. Rinse thoroughly with warm water afterwards to get rid of any residue, which can weigh your hair down or make it look straggly.

HAIR MASQUES

Hair masques have a more intensive nourishing effect than conditioners. You can now find treatments for all hair types, tailored to the condition of your hair and scalp. They contain moisturizing and lipid balancing ingredients, and some also contain silicone for sleek-feeling hair. The important thing when choosing the right hair treatment is that it suits the current state of your hair. A hair masque should always be massaged into towel-dried hair and left to work for the time specified on the pack. Please don't leave it in overnight: this can cause skin reactions. If your hair is thin and quickly looks flat, you should only use a masque on the body and ends. If your hair is very stressed, you can use one several times a week. One intensive treatment per week is enough for normal hair.

LEAVE-IN TREATMENTS

As the name suggests, these are left in your hair and don't have to be rinsed out. They are practical if you don't have time for an elaborate hair-care routine in the mornings, or if your hair is fine and stressed, and needs a light product that doesn't weigh it down. Important: always use the quantity specified in the manufacturer's instructions. Less is often more, and you can always add more if needed. Of course, a leave-in treatment is no substitute for a hair masque.

HAIR OILS

Oils are one of the oldest hair care products in the world, and they are currently enjoying a real boom: almost all hair care companies now offer a hair oil. You need to decide between natural plant oils and "dry" silicone oils. Most products contain a mix of both. The advantage of this is that your hair gets the nourishment it needs, but – if used properly – the product doesn't leave you with greasy strands. You should never use too much hair oil: one to two sprays or pumps, distributed along the length and ends of your hair, are usually sufficient. Pure plant oils should be suited to your hair type. The weight of an oil is determined by the proportion of oleic acid it contains. For fine, straight hair, use light oils like wild rose, hemp, broccoli seed, jojoba, and apricot kernel oil. Heavy oils such as olive, almond, avocado, argan, and coconut are more suited to thicker, curly hair.

IS IT WORTH BEING FAITHFUL?

Been using the same shampoo for years? In hair care, it doesn't always make sense to stay faithful to a product. From time to time, the condition of your hair changes: sometimes it's dry; sometimes it tends towards split ends, or your scalp will suddenly become oily. These changes can be caused by all kinds of things. Climate, age, eating habits, and hormonal changes can all be triggers. If you notice a change in your hair structure, change your shampoo to match.

TOOLS

To create all the beautiful looks in this book, you'll need a little bit of skill, and the right styling tools. The basic tools are listed here: these little helpers will have you creating your chosen style in no time at all.

1. PADDLE BRUSH
A paddle brush will glide easily through wet hair, and its rounded bristles massage your scalp. An ideal tool for when you are blow-drying long hair.

2. REINFORCED HAIRBRUSH
Essential for the day-to-day care of long hair. Look at the brush pad: ideally, it should be made of natural rubber, with flexible nylon bristles fixed into it. These will detangle your hair without pulling it, leaving it lovely and shiny.

3. UNREINFORCED HAIRBRUSH
For a professional-looking updo, you'll need a soft, unreinforced brush with natural bristles. It will smooth the surface of your hair, tame the ends, and make it all gleam.

4. ROUND BRUSH
This brush creates soft movement, volume, and lots of shine. Different diameters can give you anything from a bit of bounce to tighter curls. The brush should ideally have natural bristles reinforced with nylon. A round brush with a ceramic core is particularly effective at distributing hairdryer heat.

5. COMB
High quality combs are made of natural rubber or horn. It's important to buy a well-made comb, with no sharp edges that can damage your hair. Wide-toothed combs are ideal for detangling wet and dry hair, and styling combs for shaping your hair.

6. HAIRPINS
Perfect for fixing updos in place. Old pins that are bent out of shape will slip out of your hair – get rid of them!

7. HAIRGRIPS
Useful for fixing individual sections of hair in place during styling, these can also be used as hair accessories.

8. HAIRBAND/HAIR ELASTIC
Transparent hairbands made of natural rubber are a must-have. If you use fabric-covered bands, find some without a metal staple, as the metal will cause hair unnecessary stress.

9. ROLLERS
Depending on the diameter (14–70mm/½in–2¾in), you can conjure up tight curls or generous waves and volume.

10. HAIRDRYER
Should be a minimum of 1000 watts, and have several heat and speed settings. A lightweight dryer with a long cable will make blow-drying easier. A styling nozzle will direct the air stream onto individual sections, and a diffuser will stop curly hair looking fluffy.

11. CURLING TONGS
These come in different diameters, for tight curls or generous waves. Look for a digital heat control, and find a model you can hold at both ends without burning your fingers.

12. STRAIGHTENERS
These can both straighten and curl your hair. Always use high-quality straighteners with variable heat settings, and a surface that protects the hair (ideally ceramic).

13. STEEL COMB
Used for dividing hair into sections – when creating updos, for example – and of course for backcombing.

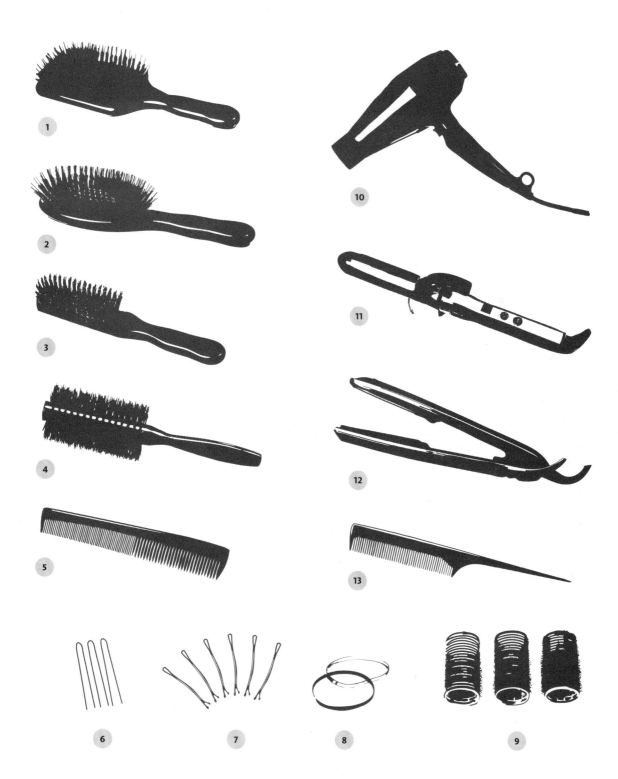

1

2

3

4

5

6

7

8

9

10

11

12

13

STYLING PRODUCTS

Blow-dry lotion, hairspray, wax, volume powder, structural spray... you can easily get lost in the jungle of styling products. Here is a brief overview of the main types of hair products, what they contain, what they do, and what special effects you can create with them.

BLOW-DRY LOTION

This has now replaced old-style setting lotion. It is mainly made up of alcohol and setting resins, and sometimes also contains nourishing ingredients like vitamins or collagen. A blow-dry lotion gives you hold and volume, and makes styling with a hairdryer and round brush easier. A good product shouldn't make your hair sticky; it should coat it with a flexible, setting film that can be brushed out. You can also get "thermoactive" blow-dry lotions, meaning that the setting effect is increased by adding heat (with a hairdryer, straighteners, or heated rollers). Use: spray the product all over towel-dried hair and give it a brief pre-blow-dry, before styling with a round or paddle brush.

STYLING MOUSSE

You can choose a styling mousse to suit your hair type. Depending on the ingredients, it can pump up fine hair, care for stressed hair or give curls more definition. It also makes your hair easier to comb and prevents it picking up a static charge. Mousse is available in various levels of hold and should not leave your hair feeling sticky. Use: depending on hair length, distribute a blob somewhere between the size of a walnut and a mandarin through your hair with a vent brush, pre-blow-dry, and shape with a brush, curling tongs, or rollers, depending on your style. For fine hair, choose a mousse that is light and airy, and not too solid, to make blow-drying easier.

HAIRSPRAY/HAIR LACQUER

This liquid hairnet consists of artificial resins, solvents, and perfumes. It protects your hair from damp conditions, wards off frizz, and gives your style more staying power. Hairspray can also be used for styling: while your hair is in rollers, for example, or sprayed on lightly while backcombing. Extra-strong hairspray is sometimes called hair lacquer. It will give you long-lasting hold, which is useful for styles like a sleek, smooth look with your hair flat against your head. Hold the can very close to your hairline, spray generously and brush into place immediately. Hair will look "wet" and gelled. Use: hairspray can be sprayed from above onto the top layer of hair, or worked in from below for more volume. Hold the can about 20cm (8in) from your head. Hairspray should be brushed out well before washing your hair, or the resins can leave a white residue.

HAIR GEL

Gel comes in different grades of solidity. The formula is based on natural or synthetic pectins (sugar compounds). Hair gel can be used on wet or dry hair, depending on the effect you want. For a casual look, add gel to wet hair and tease into shape. After drying, curls will look sculpted and defined. For a subtle wet look on short hair, rub a little gel between your palms and brush them over the surface of your hair with light, tousling movements.

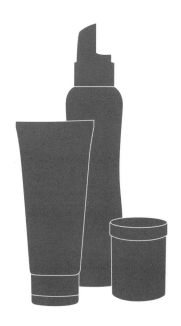

VOLUMIZING POWDER

Volumizing powder comes in little tubs, like talcum powder. It contains minerals and sugar compounds that give roots more body and hair more grip. Like mineral powder sprays, it's ideal for banishing flat roots if you have longer hair, but also perfect for styling chignons and braids. So: for more volume in your roots, shake a small (!) amount of powder onto the top of your head and work it in with your fingers. An added advantage is that the extra volume makes your hair stand away from your scalp, meaning it stays oil-free for longer. For a perfect bun or a long-lasting braid, work the volumizing powder along the length of your hair. Good to know: this magic dust always gives your hair a bit of a matte finish. If you prefer an ultra-shiny look, you should avoid volumizing powder.

STYLING CREME/HAIR WAX

Unlike hair gel, these products leave your hair soft and malleable, not solid. There are different varieties of wax and styling creme; most add shine, but some create a deliberately matte effect. Important when applying: always use the smallest possible amount to avoid weighing hair down unnecessarily. For short hair, rub a little creme or wax between your palms and run your hands through your hair with a tousling motion. If hair is longer and curly, rub styling creme or wax between your fingertips, to give the ends of your hair a high shine. If you have applied too much wax, the only remedy is to wash your hair or – if it's longer – tie it back.

HEAT PROTECTION PRODUCTS

The heat from hair dryers and the 220°C (430°F) reached by straighteners can take a lot out of your hair. Over time it becomes stressed, and can end up dry, dull, and brittle. The heat can also cause split ends and breakage. Heat protection products, in the form of sprays or gels, protect hair from this damage. They wrap a super-fine protective coat of polymers around each individual hair, shielding it from the heat. A good heat protection product should leave your hair soft and shiny, not hard or oily. Caution: the latest research shows that 185°C (365°F) is the optimum temperature for styling hair without damaging it. High-quality devices will have a temperature regulator.

STRUCTURE SPRAY

A relatively new addition to the styling product market. Structure sprays, also called micro powder sprays and mineral fixing sprays, contain the mineral salt calcium carbonate, together with a fixing polymer. The mineral salt has a texturizing effect, giving your hair a kind of matte, sugar-water look, though without leaving it feeling rough. This makes it easier to backcomb. Structure sprays can give updos more volume and better structure, and styles last better because your hair is less slippery. Important: shake the spray well before use and spray onto roots for added volume. For shorter hair, you can also use the spray on the body and ends for a wilder look.

MORE BOUNCE FOR YOUR CURLS

For a while now, a range of products have been available specifically for curls and waves. They contain ingredients that give hair a lot of moisture – and keep it there. This makes your hair less frizzy, gives it a lovely shine, and curls look tighter and more defined. These products don't make hair hard or sticky, and curls should stay soft and flexible.

TIMELESS BEAUTY: CLASSIC HAIRSTYLES

Here they are: the classic hairstyles. They've been in fashion for decades, and are always being adapted to current trends. Starting with these four basic cuts, you can conjure up styles to suit every type and face shape.

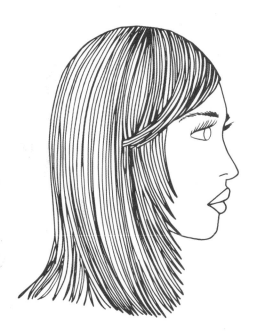 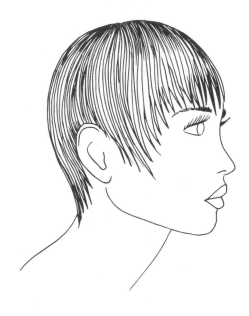

LOVELY LAYERS: THE SHAG

Jane Fonda inspired people with this layered cut back in the 1970s. Meg Ryan gave us the short version, which has been copied countless times by women all over the world. The shag is basically a layered style, cut close to the head. It can be worn at almost any length – from above the jawline to shoulder-length (also called a clavicut). Its trademark is a soft, cheeky side-fringe, which falls over the forehead. Styling is easy: wash and blow-dry, tousle with your fingers, and work in some styling creme – that's all it needs. This cut looks best with straight hair, or hair with some natural, gentle movement. It isn't suitable for tight curls.

IN SHORT: THE GARÇON CUT

Of course, you need a bit of courage for a radical, short haircut. But the appeal of the short garçon-style cut lies in the relatively long top hair, with feathered sides falling softly over the temples and leaving the ears exposed. It can be worn with a side parting or a choppy fringe. Styling this look couldn't be easier: leave your hair to air dry, or give it a quick blast with a hairdryer, then rub a little wax between your palms and use it to bring the hair forwards towards your face. Good to know: if you go for an extreme look like this, you will have to do a little more with your make up. Bright red lips or strong, smoky eyes provide a feminine contrast to a slightly boyish haircut. Pretty stud earrings or larger hoops also go well with this style.

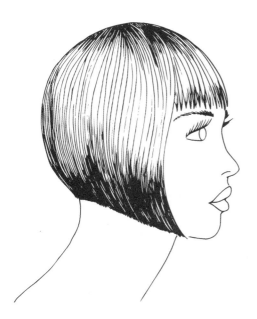

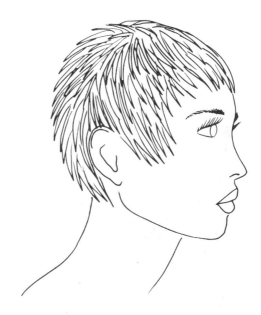

GEOMETRIC AND SHINY: THE BOB

The bob, or page-boy cut, was a modern look in ancient Egypt. It underwent a big revival in the 1920s. And when the Beatles came on the scene with their mop tops, the cut became a symbol for a rebellious generation. Precise, geometric contours are important for a bob. The cut has many variants: all the hair can be worn at the same length, but the interesting variations are those with a shorter, graduated back, as in the drawing above. Length-wise, anything is possible from earlobes to collarbone (lob = long bob), and asymmetric bobs look great, too. They are usually worn with a full fringe, but a choppier front or side fringe look good as well.

SOFT AND LAYERED: THE PIXIE

Stars like Jean Seberg or Mia Farrow brought the pixie to Hollywood in the 1960s. As the name suggests, the cut has a cheeky, elfin edge. Unlike the garçon cut, the hair is layered all over, and looks relatively feminine despite its short length. The short cut will be at its very best if your hair has a natural, light wave. It's easy to style: blow-dry, rub a little wax or styling creme between your palms, and work it into your hair with your fingers. This will give it the necessary structure. You can go for more dramatic make-up with a pixie cut, especially to emphasize your eyes.

CHANGING FRINGES

There are plenty of good reasons to have a fringe: it can emphasize beautiful eyes, conceal a high forehead, give many haircuts a cheeky edge, and even distract from fine lines. But all fringes are not equal. It's amazing what effects you can achieve with different varieties...

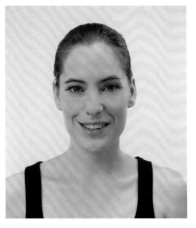

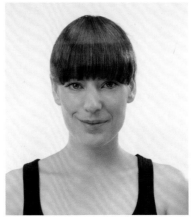

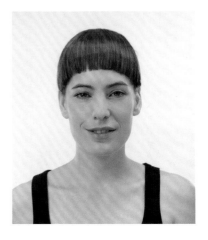

NO FRINGE
Our model with her hair combed back, revealing a lovely oval face, with large eyes and a relatively large forehead. Your gaze is particularly drawn to her mouth.

LONG
A very long, very full fringe improves the proportions of the face and emphasizes the eyes in particular. Tip: blow-dry using a large round brush.

TRENDY
An ultra-short, trendy fringe requires courage: it's like adding an exclamation mark to your style. Emphasized eyebrows are important for this look. Styling: straighten with hair straighteners.

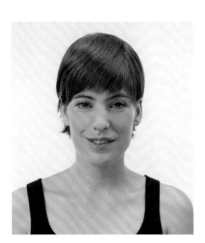

CHEEKY
A choppy, not-too-short side fringe looks casual and not at all preppy. Tousle with your fingers while blow-drying, and work in a blob of styling creme.

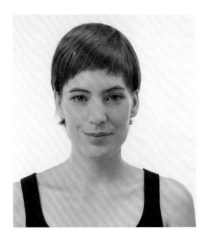

GARÇON-LIKE
A round-cut, choppy short fringe looks a bit boyish, but still not too severe. A quick blow-dry, and you're good to go.

PERFECT PARTINGS

Whether it's a Madonna-style centre parting, a classic side parting or an extravagant zig-zag look: styling your parting lets you whip up a whole new effect for your style, especially if you have longer hair.

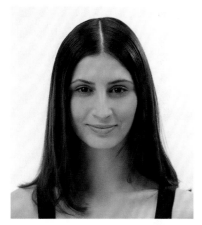

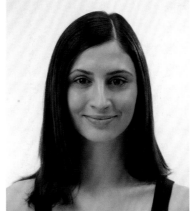

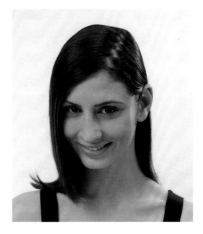

ELEGANT
A centre parting will give you a classy look. It emphasizes the face, so your features should be symmetrical. Caution: this will make narrow faces look even narrower.

CLASSIC
A side parting suits most women. It can emphasize your best side and attract attention away from the other. As you part your hair, check the shape it makes around your face.

SOMETHING SPECIAL
For a zig-zag parting, comb your hair back from your face and hold with one hand. Use a steel comb to draw a zig-zag line from front to back.

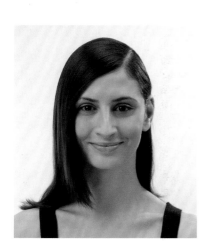

ON TREND
A very low side parting will conceal a high forehead and lengthen a round face. Try giving one side a wet look, styled tight against your head.

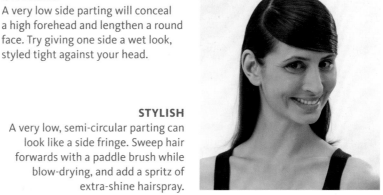

STYLISH
A very low, semi-circular parting can look like a side fringe. Sweep hair forwards with a paddle brush while blow-drying, and add a spritz of extra-shine hairspray.

THE LOOKS

Wearable and fashionable, elegant and stylish:
these are special looks you can wear every day.

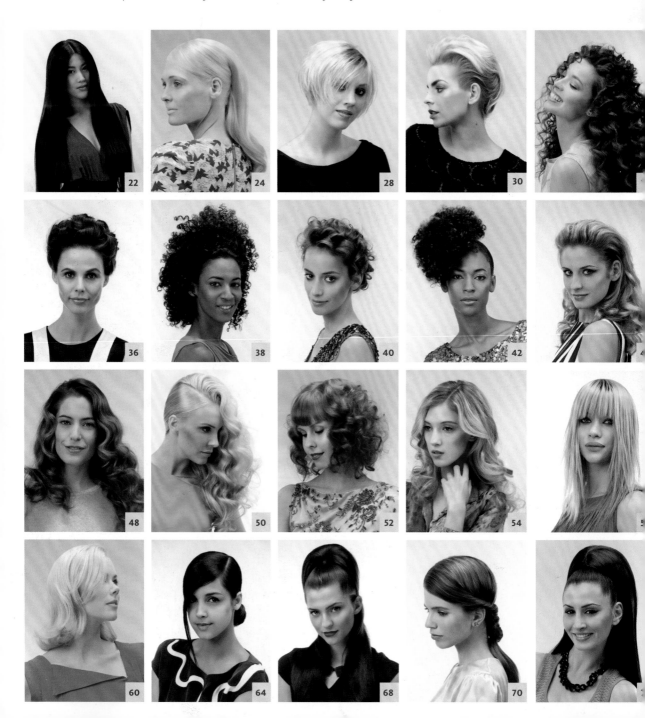

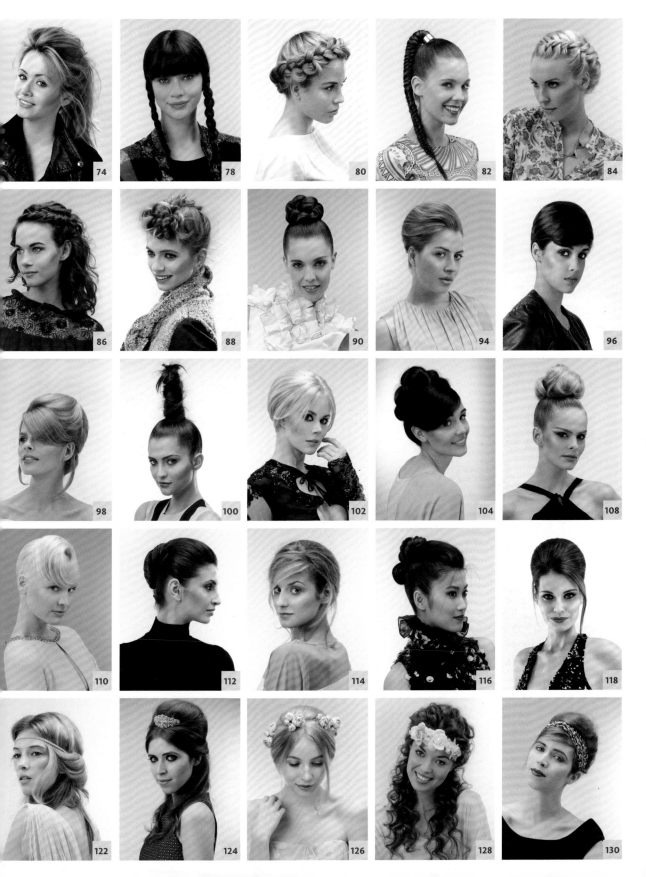

74

78

80

82

84

86

88

90

94

96

98

100

102

104

108

110

112

114

116

118

122

124

126

128

130

VOLUME

Who doesn't want a bit more body in their hair? The key to achieving volume is a perfect cut, along with some clever styling tricks that can turn even fine hair into a luxurious mane.

ROUND BRUSH

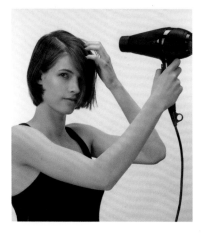 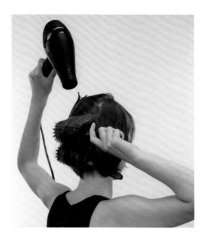

1. DRY
Comb out freshly washed hair, work in some setting lotion and pre-dry well with a hairdryer. If your hair is too damp, styling it will take a long time.

2. ROLL
Divide your hair into not-too-thick sections. Clip the hair you're not styling out of the way. The diameter of the brush will determine how much volume you can achieve.

3. BLOW-DRY
Styling will be much quicker if you work with several round brushes at the same time. As you're drying a new section, the previous one can be left on the brush to cool.

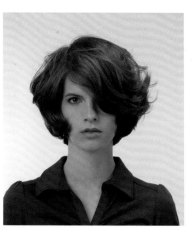 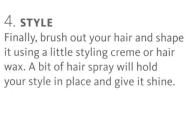

4. STYLE
Finally, brush out your hair and shape it using a little styling creme or hair wax. A bit of hair spray will hold your style in place and give it shine.

SHINE AND BODY

To create beautiful shine, pull a round brush through your hair to the tips, being careful not to fold the ends over as you turn it. Work with, not against, gravity – tilting your head to the side or the front as you blow-dry. To create volume in your roots, pre-dry them thoroughly before starting, otherwise the moisture there will work its way into the rest of your hair and your style will collapse or go frizzy. If possible, leave the brush in your hair to cool. Alternatively, clip the blow-dried sections in place, or use rollers.

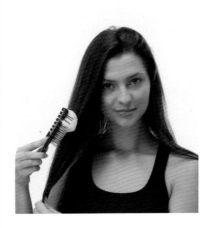

1. BRUSH IN

Put some styling or setting mousse on a vent brush or hairbrush and work it into your hair from roots to tips.

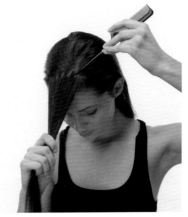

2. DIVIDE

Use a steel comb to divide your hair into equal, not-too-large sections, along zig-zag lines. Start creating your volume with the top front section.

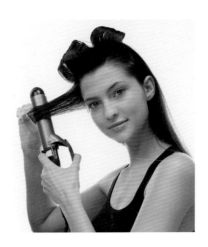

3. WRAP

Wrap one section at a time around your chosen size of curling tongs. Be careful not to fold the ends over, and clip each curl to the top of your head as you go.

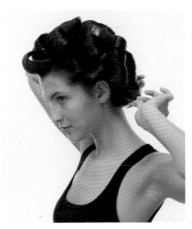

4. FIX

Carry on until all your hair is curled. Leave the curls clipped up until they are completely cool – this will ensure really good hold and elasticity.

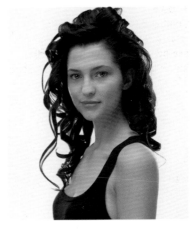

5. FINISH

Once your hair is cool, carefully remove the clips, brush out with a styling brush, and loosen with your hands. A spritz of hairspray will give you even more body.

MEGA MANES

Very long, thick hair is so heavy it can sometimes lose a bit of volume at the roots. But the right styling products and a neat backcombing trick will give your long locks more body.

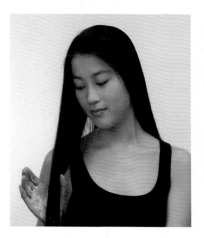

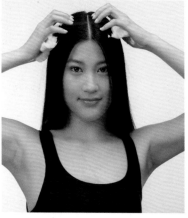

SILKY SHINE
Very long hair can often lose its shine, as the lengths and ends get older over the years, and go through various stresses. A shine spray provides a quick solution. Spray very sparingly (!) onto hair; its combination of natural and silicone oils will give you a lovely instant gleam.

1. SMOOTH
To give hair a beautiful shine, smooth the body and ends of your hair with a little styling cream. Rub the cream between your palms, and run them through your hair.

2. ADD MOUSSE
For more volume on top, massage a golf-ball-sized amount of mousse into your roots with both hands. For thermoactive products, give your hair a quick blast with a hairdryer.

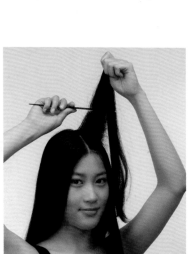

3. BACKCOMB
Lift the hair in sections with your hand and backcomb using a steel comb. Then brush through the surface hair with a hairdresser's brush to make the hair smooth again.

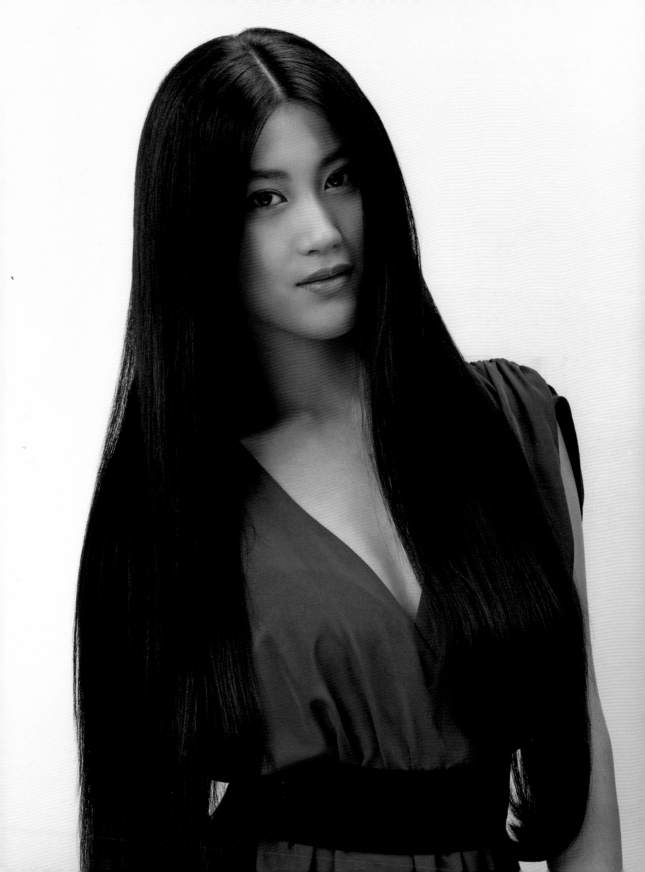

VOLUME TWIST WITH IMPACT

Platinum blonde hair suits a stand-out look, and this style is futuristic and very cool. The updo variation, with a coil of hair pinned to the back of your head, gives the whole thing a classical Roman touch.

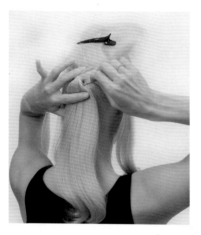

1. DIVIDE
Make a horizontal parting with a comb below your crown, from ear to ear, and tie back the lower section into a high ponytail with a transparent hairband.

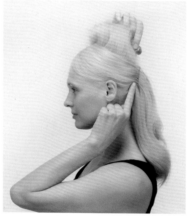

2. FIX
Make a low, short side parting and sweep your hair around the sides of your head, fixing it at the back on each side of the ponytail.

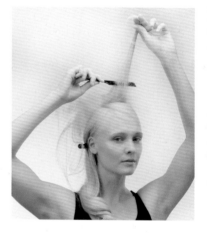

3. BACKCOMB
Thoroughly backcomb the middle section on the top of your head with a steel comb. A little structural spray will give hair much more grip and make it easier to style.

HOW TO BACKCOMB
Holding a section of hair by the ends, insert a steel comb close to the roots and pull down several times against the direction of growth. The individual hairs will mesh together, giving hair more grip and volume. Important: if you are backcombing every day, you will need some intensive hair care.

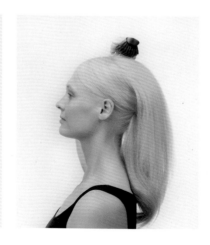

4. BRUSH SMOOTH
Use a styling brush to brush the surface of the backcombed hair smooth, and let it fall over the pinned sections on the back of your head. Fix in place with hairspray.

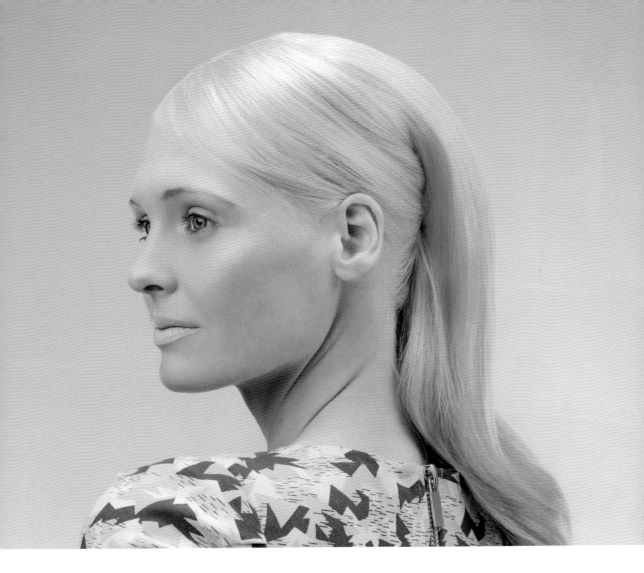

*Variation: twist
the ponytail into
a loose coil and
pin it in place.
The ends should
remain visible.*

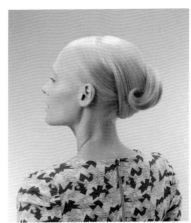

AN ADAPTABLE PIXIE CUT

Short, but anything but boring: that's the best way to describe the classic pixie. Don't be fooled into thinking that its length means there's no room for change. Here are the prettiest variations on the timeless short cut.

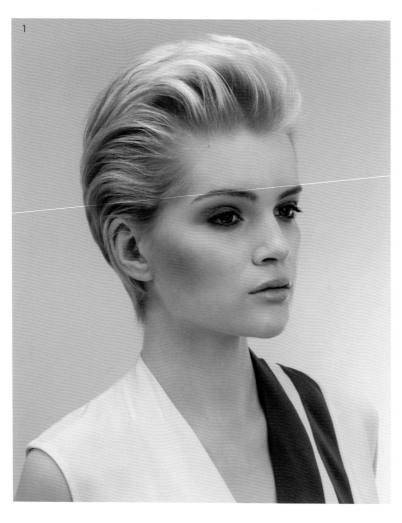

1

1. ELEGANT

Styled completely out of the face, this pixie looks sophisticated and glamorous, and has what it takes for a really elegant evening look. Here's how to style it: work some styling mousse or setting spray into damp hair, and brush it towards the back of your head with a vent or paddle brush as you blow-dry. Rub a little styling creme between your palms and style the sides back close against your head. You can also give the front section a quick backcomb for more volume. Set in place with lots of hairspray.

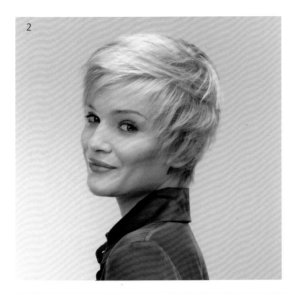

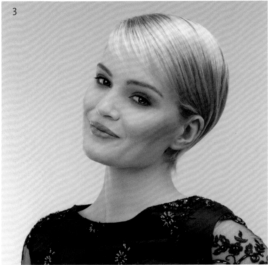

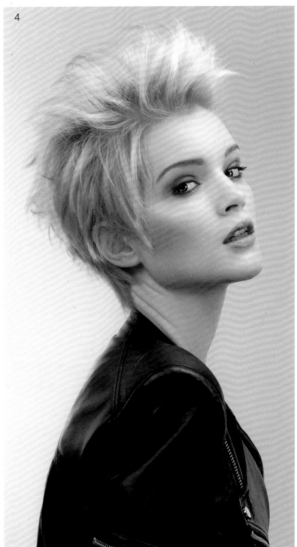

2. TOUSLED

This is a casual, cheeky look – and it's incredibly easy to style, even if you're pushed for time in the morning. Blow-dry your hair, directing the air forwards, backwards, right, and left alternately. Rub a little hair wax between your palms and run your hands through your hair to tousle it.

3. SLEEK

A great, fashionable style that will take you from day to evening. Here's how: use a paddle brush to blow-dry hair smooth and flat against your head (for hair with some natural bounce, you can apply a smoothing product beforehand). Rub a little styling creme between your palms and stroke them over your hair.

4. PUNKY

Every woman should be a bit of a rebel now and then. Turn your pixie into a wild, rocky cut. Styling is easy: distribute some setting mousse through your hair and blow-dry. Thoroughly backcomb the middle section on top of your head with a steel comb, adding structural spray as you go for extra volume. Fix in place with hairspray.

UNSTRUCTURED MINI BOB

This look is based on a layered, ear-length bob. Our example shows how much variety a short cut can give you – and with hair this length, styling takes no time at all.

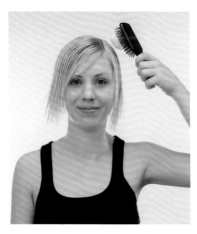

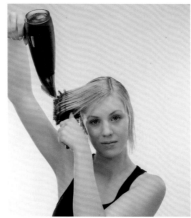

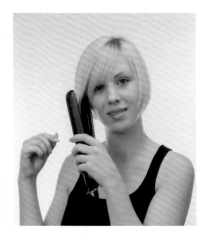

1. BRUSH IN
Squeeze a golf-ball-sized amount of styling mousse onto a paddle brush, and brush through towel-dried hair from root to tip.

2. BLOW-DRY
Pre-dry your hair with a hairdryer. When it's almost dry, start using a large round brush – this will give your hair a lovely shine.

3. STRAIGHTEN
Apply a heat-protection product to the ends of your hair before straightening it, turning the straighteners inwards slightly as you go. Tousle with your hands to finish.

PLAYING WITH COLOUR
A great hair colour with lots of shine can really bring a bob into its own. On blonde hair, different tones will loosen up your style. Caution: lowlights – darker strands – can quickly look dirty in blonde hair. Leaving darker roots will give hair more depth and make it appear fuller.

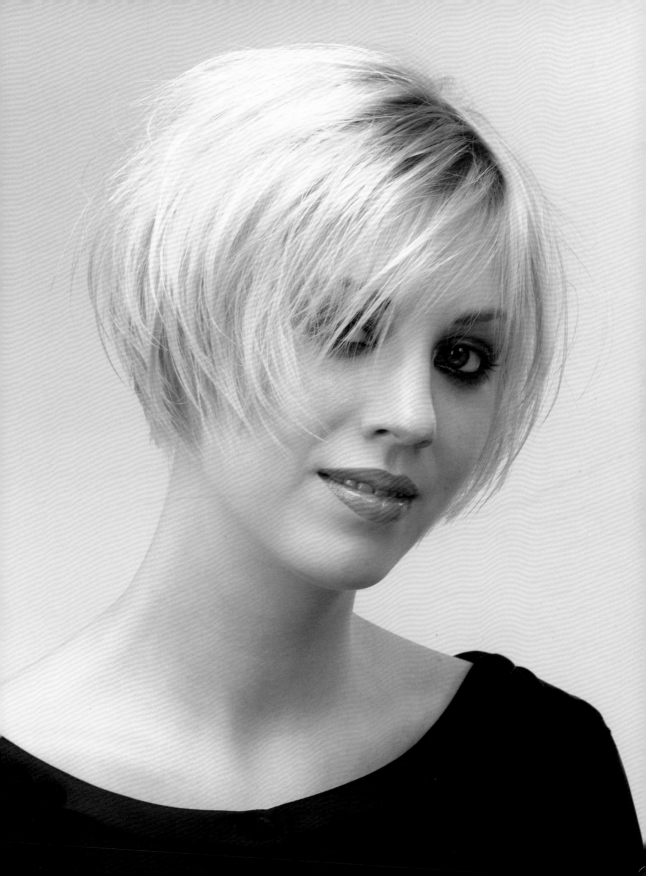

FLOWING UPDO

A contrasting look: from the front and side, this updo almost gives the impression of being an androgynous short cut, but from the back it looks soft and feminine.

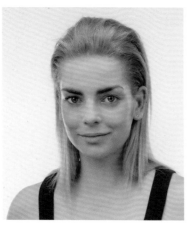

1. PREPARE
For this look, hair should be at least shoulder length, and can be straight or wavy. Comb the front section back off your forehead, and brush the rest of your hair smooth.

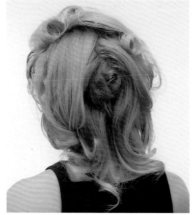

2. PIN UP
Backcomb a not-too-thin section at the back of your head, roll it up with your fingers and use two crossed hair grips to pin it into a mini knot. This will serve as a cushion.

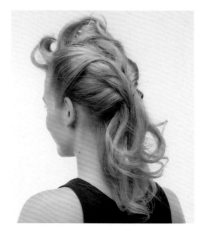

3. DRAPE
Divide the rest of your hair into strands and pin them to the cushion knot with hair pins, as invisibly as possible. Your hair should hang straight down from the centre.

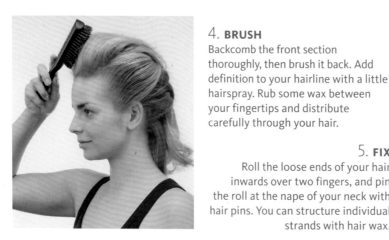

4. BRUSH
Backcomb the front section thoroughly, then brush it back. Add definition to your hairline with a little hairspray. Rub some wax between your fingertips and distribute carefully through your hair.

5. FIX
Roll the loose ends of your hair inwards over two fingers, and pin the roll at the nape of your neck with hair pins. You can structure individual strands with hair wax.

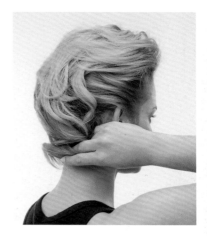

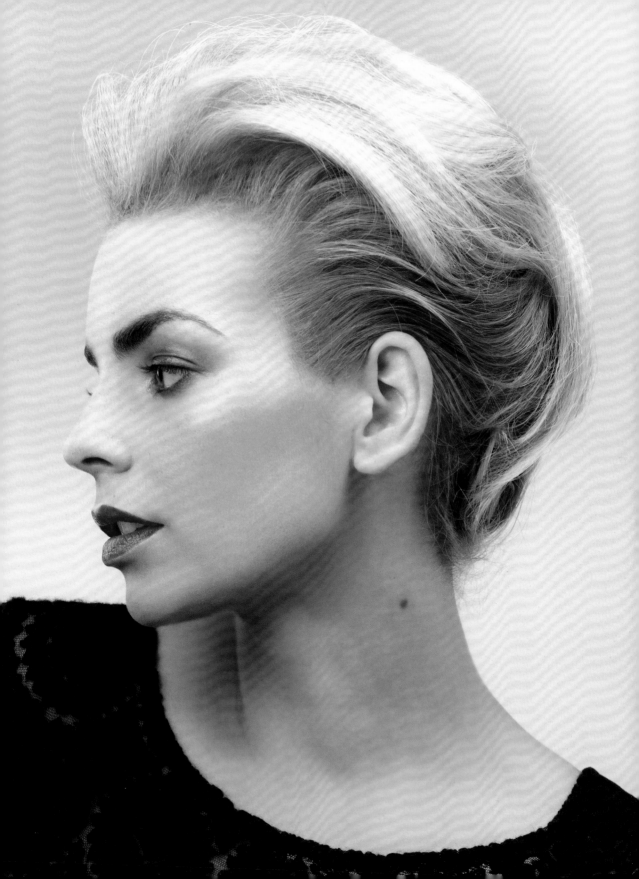

CURLS

From soft and romantic to a casual, unstructured look: curls flatter the face and suit everyone. With these techniques, the waves you want will be literally at your fingertips.

FINGER TWIST WITH HAIRCLIPS

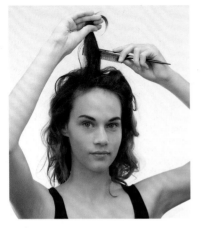

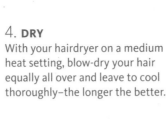

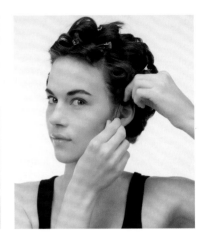

1. DIVIDE
One at a time, separate out relatively thin strands with a steel comb, spray with blow-dry lotion and comb through so that the product covers the whole length of the strand.

2. TWIST
Use your fingers to twist each strand around itself, and then around two fingers, into a not-too-tight curl. Clip the curl in place with a hairclip.

3. FIX
Repeat this process with the rest of your hair until all the strands have been curled and clipped to your head. Spray more blow-dry lotion over the whole thing.

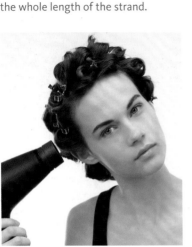

4. DRY
With your hairdryer on a medium heat setting, blow-dry your hair equally all over and leave to cool thoroughly—the longer the better.

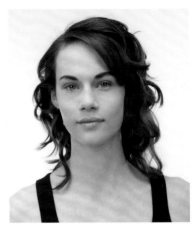

5. SHAPE
One by one, carefully take out the hair clips. Don't brush the curls out; just tease them out individually with your fingers.

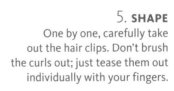

OVERNIGHT CURLS

You can even conjure up the waves you want in your sleep. For "rag" curls, curl your hair around cosmetic or paper tissues folded lengthways, and leave overnight. First, dampen hair with a little blow-dry spray or hairspray. Make a centre parting that starts at the nape of your neck, and wrap two sections on either side around tissues, knotting the ends when they are wrapped. Do the same with four more sections at the front and above the ears. Take out in the morning and comb out carefully. A spritz of hairspray and you're good to go!

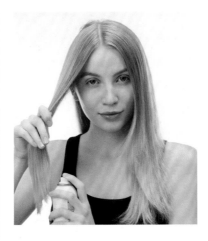

1. PREPARE

Make a side parting and separate your hair into four large sections. Cover these one at a time with plenty of extra-strong hairspray.

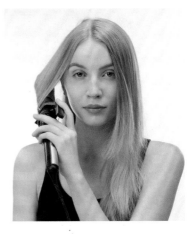

2. CURL

Curl each wide section of hair around large-barrelled curling tongs. Be careful not to fold the ends of your hair under when curling, as this will make the end result less attractive.

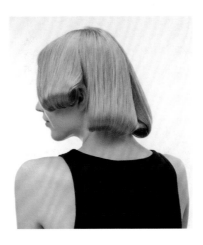

3. COOL

Secure these large curls to their roots, using several hairgrips for each, and leave to cool thoroughly. The longer you leave them, the longer your look will last.

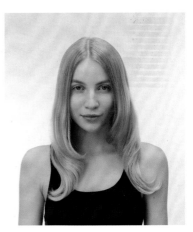

4. STYLE

When they are completely cool, carefully remove the clips and brush into shape for soft curls, or just shape with your fingers for structured, corkscrew curls.

LUXURIOUS CURLS

If you have straight hair, you long for curls, and women with waves dream of a sleek look. That's just the way it is. This super twist lets you transform even ultra-straight hair into natural-looking spiral curls, one strand at a time.

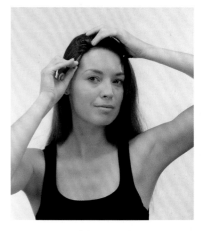

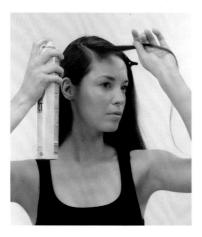

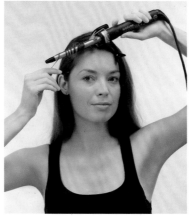

1. SPRAY
Give yourself a side parting and spray a thin strand of hair with enough hairspray to give it a slight damp sheen. Clip your remaining hair to one side for easier working.

2. CURL
Twist the sprayed strand around itself, before carefully wrapping it around small-barrelled curling tongs.

3. CLIP
Remove the curling tongs very carefully, holding the curl in place with your hand, and clip it securely to your head.

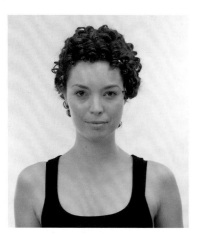

4. DRY
Carry on until all your hair is twisted in thin strands and clipped up. Only move on to the next step once the last curl is completely cool.

5. UNCLIP
Once your hair is cool, remove the clips. Be careful not to brush your hair afterwards; just tease it out with your fingers to retain the structure of the curls.

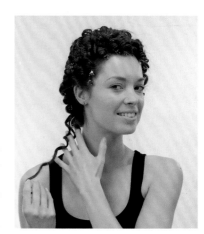

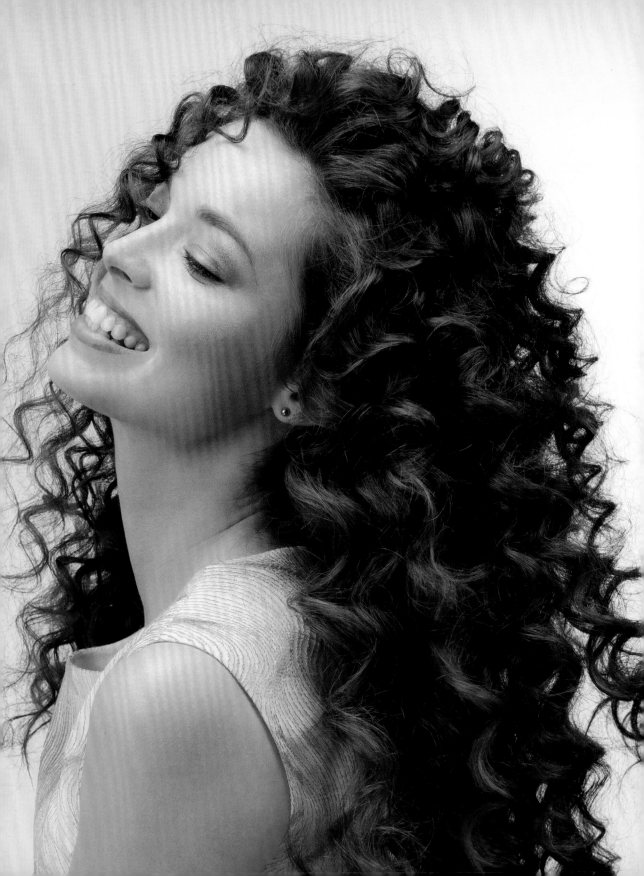

UPDO WITH CURLS

This style is great if your hair is at least shoulder-length. It's an updo with a difference: small sections are rolled into soft curls with your fingers and pinned on top of your head. Very feminine – and extremely glamorous.

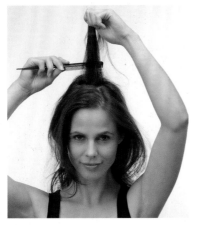

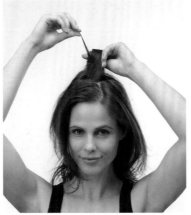

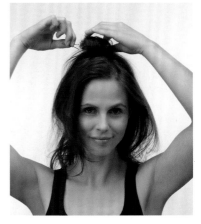

1. BACKCOMB
Give yourself a side parting. Take a relatively thin strand from the top of your head and backcomb it thoroughly. If your hair is very soft, add a little structure spray.

2. ROLL
Roll the backcombed section around two fingers. Make sure the roll isn't too tight, and take care to avoid folding the ends. Hold it in place with the other hand as you carefully take your fingers out.

3. PIN
Fix the roll in place with several hairgrips or pins. Make sure they disappear into the hair, and the roll isn't pressed flat.

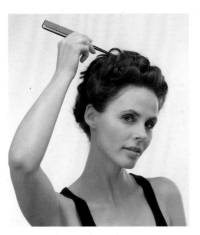

4. LOOSEN
Roll up the rest of your hair section by section, as described in steps 1–3. Finally, lift and loosen the curls a little with the end of a steel comb.

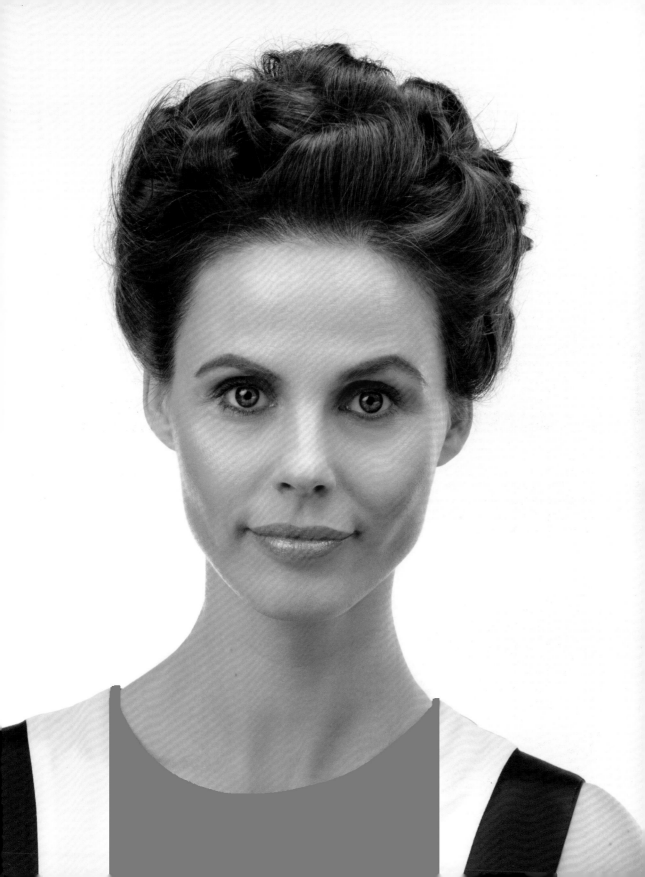

AFRO VOLUME

The typical problem for Afro curls and naturally frizzy hair is that your hair can look like an undefined mass. But you can combat the candyfloss look. Diffusors and styling products will tame and define your roots.

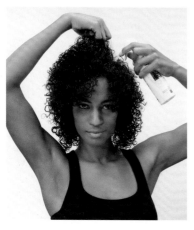

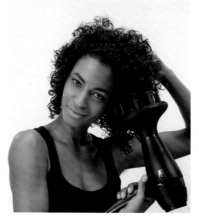

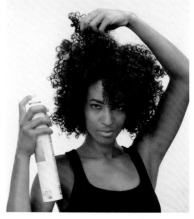

1. SET
After washing, spray a thermoactive blow-dry spray into damp hair. This will create volume, shine and structure, and protect your hair from dryer heat.

2. DRY
Blow-dry your hair using a diffusor attachment. Holding it against your hair stops your curls fluffing up in the air stream.

3. LOOSEN
Lift individual sections with your fingers and spray a bit of hairspray or lacquer onto them from underneath, creating volume where you want it.

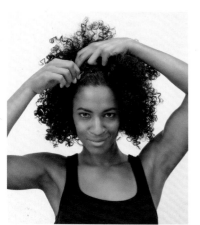

4. PIN
Brush the front section of your hair back from your forehead and pin it down with hairgrips two finger-widths from your hairline. Fix in place with hairspray, then remove the pins.

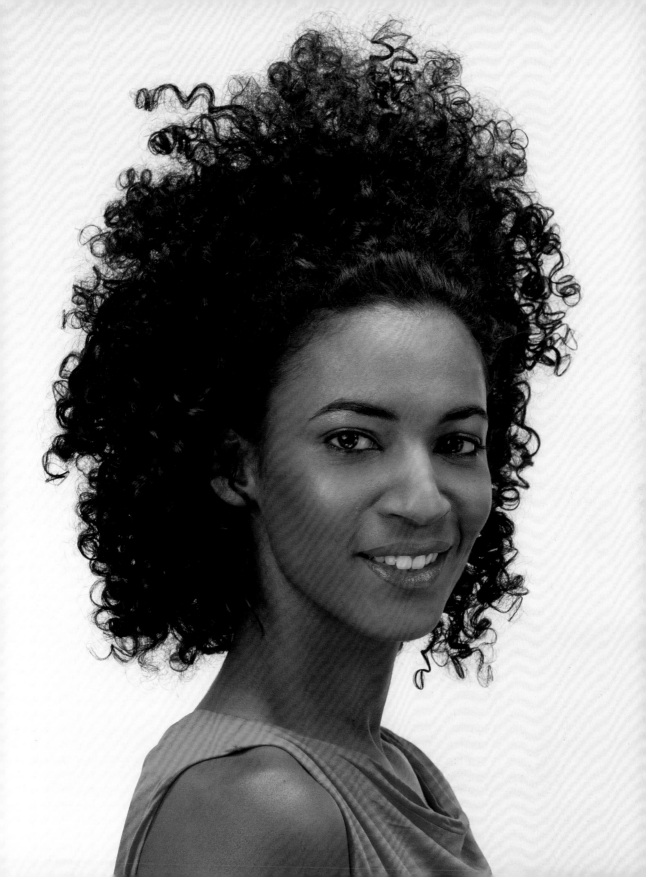

CURLED CHIGNON

Want a soft, feminine, romantic style? Then try this combination of a bun and gentle curls. The curls take a little bit of time, but the results are worth it!

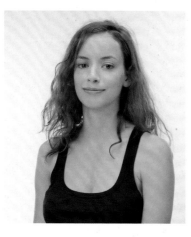

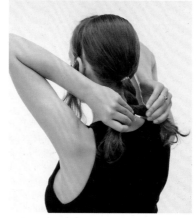

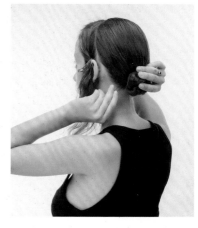

1. PREPARE
This style is perfect for at least shoulder length hair. Your hair structure doesn't matter, but if you have natural curls you can save time by skipping the curling step.

2. TIE
Pin two large side sections of hair out of the way with clips. Tie the rest of your hair into a ponytail, separate it into two strands, twist these together and tie off with a hairband.

3. KNOT
Roll the twisted ponytail into a round bun on the nape of your neck. Pin it securely in place with hairpins, trying not to let these show.

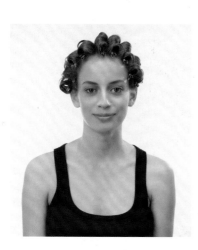

4. CURL
Spray the side sections with hairspray, then curl thin strands over your middle finger and clip them up. After ten minutes, remove the clips and tease out the curls with your fingers.

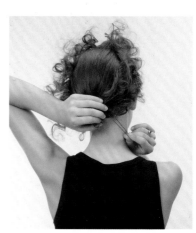

5. FIX
Gently sweep the curly front sections back and pin them loosely around the bun.

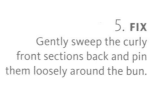

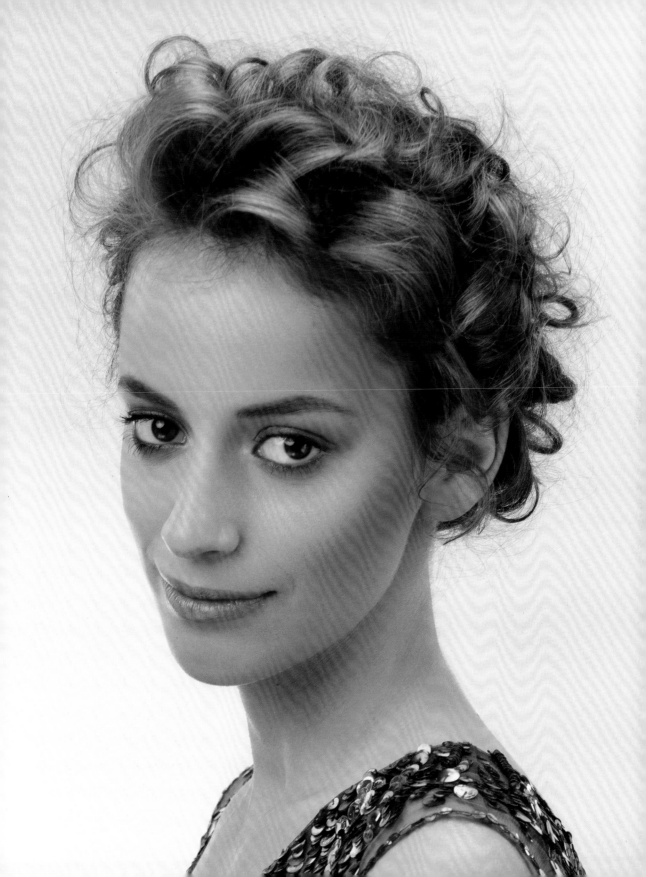

SIDE POMPADOUR

Tight natural curls or a genuine Afro can be difficult to tame. Here is an updo that makes a true feature of your curls – and is simple enough to manage even when you don't have much time.

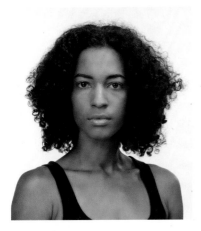

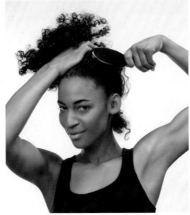

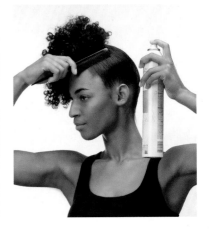

1. PREPARE
The pompadour is ideal for chin to shoulder-length hair. If your hair is much longer, you will need more hairpins to turn it into a pompadour.

2. BRUSH UP
Brush all your hair over to one side of the top of your head, and tie it into a high ponytail using a transparent hairband.

3. SMOOTH
Create a wet look by spraying a lot of hairspray onto your hair and smoothing it down with a styling comb. This will make even very curly hair look sleek.

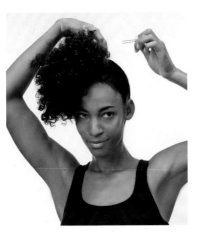

4. FIX
Use a few hairpins to shape the pompadour on the front of your head, making it round and not too high.

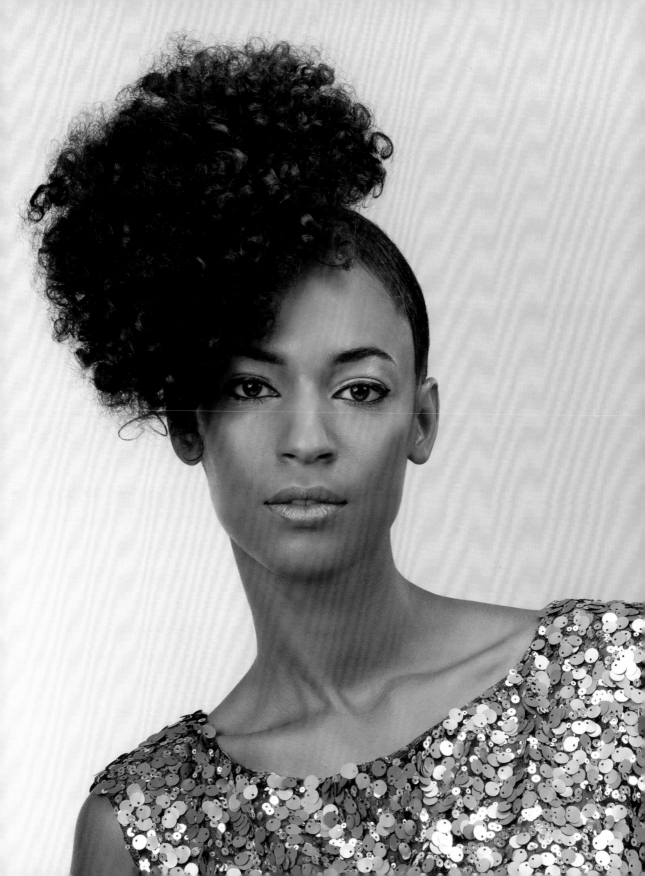

SOFT CURLS WITH VOLUME

Big hair never really goes out of fashion. This style combines soft, natural waves with volume on the top of your head. The result is a very feminine look with a touch of Hollywood glamour.

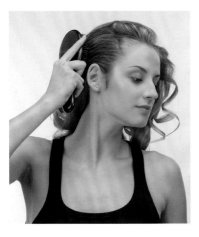

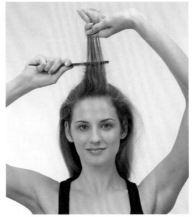

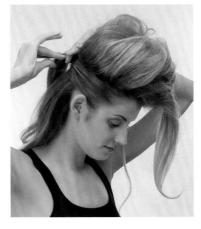

1. BRUSH FLAT
Brush the side sections of your hair firmly back from your temples using a styling brush, using lots of hairspray as you go for hold and shine – it should create a slight wet look.

2. BACKCOMB
Backcomb the remaining top front section of hair thoroughly. Add structure spray for extra volume, and to ensure your hair doesn't collapse.

3. BRING TOGETHER
Take the brushed-back sections from Step 1 and tie them together at the back of your head with a transparent hairband. Let the backcombed section of your hair fall over it.

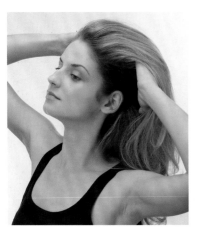

4. LOOSEN
Put both hands into the outer layers of your hair and loosen up the style a little with a gentle tousling motion. Add some hairspray or lacquer to finish.

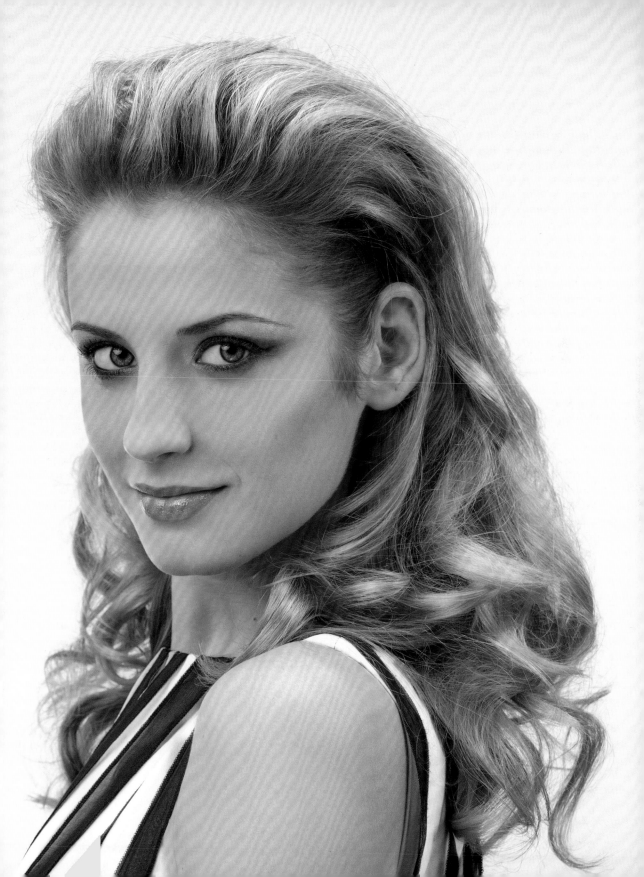

BASIC TECHNIQUES
WAVES

Looking for gentle, generous glamour waves or a hippyish, crimped style? Different styling techniques will help you create a mind-boggling variety of wavy looks.

ROLLERS

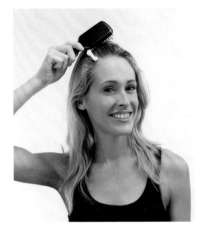 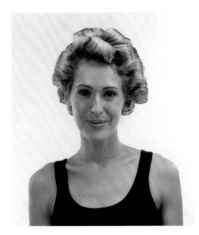

1. PREPARE
Add a little styling mousse to a paddle or vent brush, and brush it through wet or dry hair from roots to tips.

2. ROLL
Starting with the top front section, wrap your hair around your chosen size of roller. Use a steel comb to make sure the tips don't get folded under.

3. DRY
Do the same with the side sections, and then the hair at the back of your head, until all your hair is in rollers. Blow-dry thoroughly with a hairdryer or hood dryer.

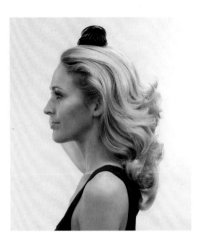

4. BRUSH OUT
Important: leave hair to cool well – this will help your waves last longer. Remove the rollers and brush your hair back, starting from your forehead, to shape it. Hairspray will hold your style in place.

ROCK AND ROLL

Self-grip or Velcro rollers come in different sizes, from 12mm (½in) minis to jumbo rollers 73mm (2¾in) in diameter. The basic rule is: the larger the roller, the softer and larger your waves will be. The very small ones let you create curls and ringlets. Important when rolling: comb out each strand well before use so that hairs don't get tangled in the fine plastic hooks. Always roll the tips cleanly and be careful not to rip out any hairs as you roll.

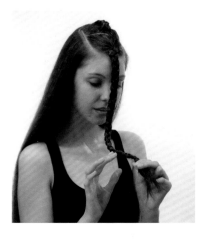

1. BRAID

Make two partings in your hair to divide it into three sections. Starting at the front, braid a thick strand and tie the end with a hairband.

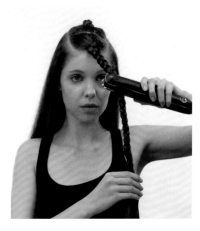

2. REINFORCE

Heat the braid one section at a time with straighteners, applying gentle pressure. The heat reinforces the crimped structure that the braids will give you.

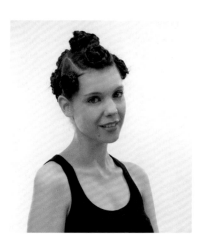

3. TWIST

Carry on until you have around eight to ten braided and heated sections. Twist each braid into a coil and fix it to your head with hairgrips.

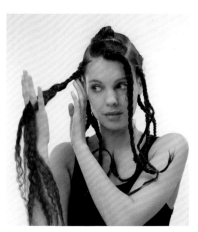

4. TAKE OUT

Ideally you should keep the braids in overnight, but a few hours during the day is fine too. Remove the grips and hairbands, and gently tease out the braids with your fingers.

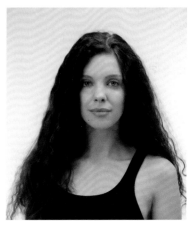

5. STYLE

Don't brush or comb your hair, as this will destroy the structure. Just shape it using your fingers and a little styling creme or hair wax.

WILD WAVES

Want generous, glamorous waves, not cute baby-doll curls?
You can get this look without chemical setting, even if your hair
is completely straight. The trick is to use curling tongs with the
right-sized barrel, and the right setting method.

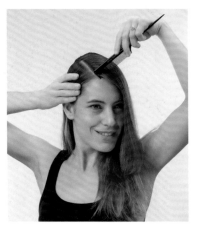

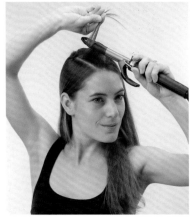

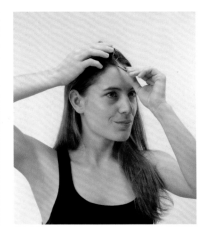

1. DIVIDE
This look is ideal for long hair, starting at about shoulder length. First, make an accurate side parting and separate a relatively thin strand from the front section.

2. WAVE
Spray on some heat protection or hairspray and wrap the strand around medium-barrelled curling tongs. Be very careful as you wrap the ends.

3. PIN
Hold the curl in place as you carefully remove the curling tongs, and pin it up with a hairgrip. Use the same method to roll the rest of your hair.

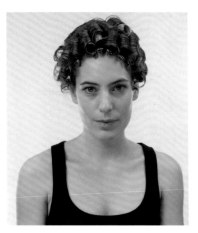

4. WAIT
When all your hair is curled and pinned in place, wait until it's completely cool, and then carefully remove the grips, one by one.

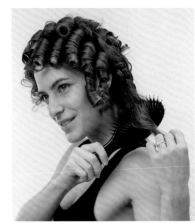

5. BRUSH OUT
Starting at the nape of your neck, hold the end of each strand gently as you run a brush through it. Finally, give your hair a little shake out.

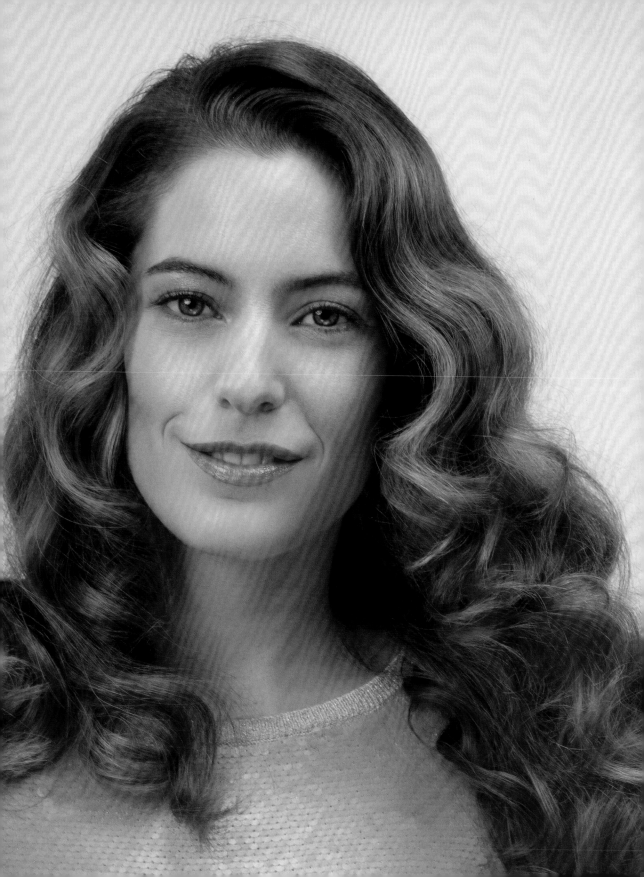

SIDE-SWEEP WITH CURLS

An asymmetrical style is always something a bit special. It will make your hair look completely different from every angle, and emphasize your best side. This curled side-sweep look is pure Hollywood glamour.

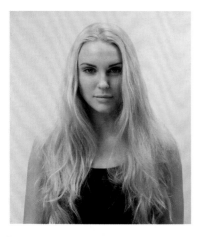

1. PART
Your hair should be at least shoulder-length for this look, and it doesn't matter if it's straight: curling tongs will provide the glamour waves. Make a side parting.

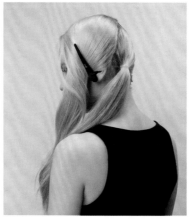

2. SEPARATE
Brush your hair to one side and tie half of it into a ponytail behind your ear. Dividing up the rest with a large hair clip makes it easier to work with the curling tongs.

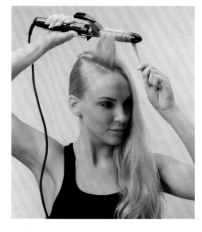

3. CURL
One at a time, wrap thin strands from the loose side around the curling tongs, not too tightly. Then carefully remove the tongs, and pin the curl up with a hairgrip.

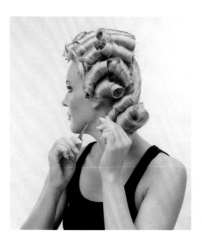

4. CLIP
Carry on until all the strands are rolled into curls and clipped up. For a longer hold, leave them to cool thoroughly, then remove the clips and brush through.

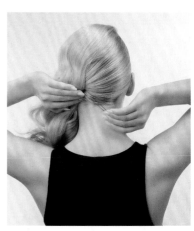

5. FIX
Pin the curled side in place with hairpins, low on the back of your head, keeping the pins as invisible as possible. Fix well with hairspray.

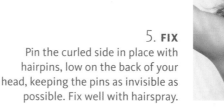

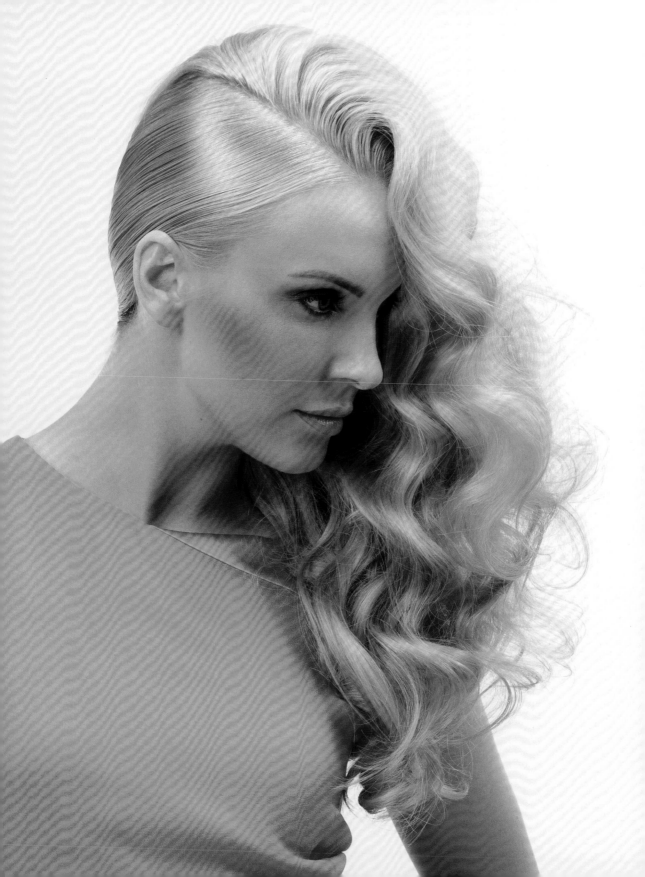

WAVES WITH CONTRAST

Naturally wavy hair isn't easy to style, and can end up looking the same whatever you do. Here is the solution for creating a bit of variety, with free-flowing curls and a straight fringe – and this style makes shoulder-length hair chin-length.

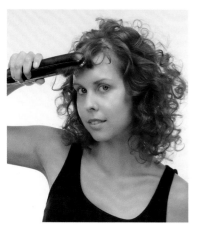

1. STRAIGHTEN
Divide your fringe into two or three sections and straighten it with hair straighteners, using a light pressure. Important: apply a heat-protection product before starting.

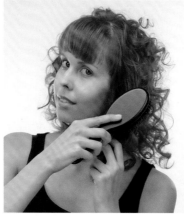

2. BRUSH OUT
Brush out your curls with a styling brush, smoothing your hair with your hand after every stroke. You can fix it with some extra-strong hairspray.

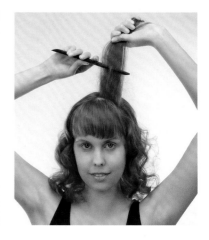

3. BACKCOMB
Lightly backcomb your roots to give the style more volume. Brush the surface hair smooth again, and add a little hairspray to the roots.

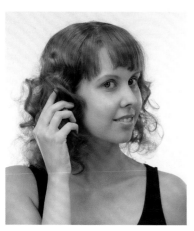

4. SHAPE
Use your hands to shape your curls into waves. Take individual sections in your hand and scrunch gently to give the waves more structure.

5. PIN
Tie the back section of your hair into a low ponytail with a transparent hairband. Turn the end of the ponytail under, and pin it in place as invisibly as you can with hairpins.

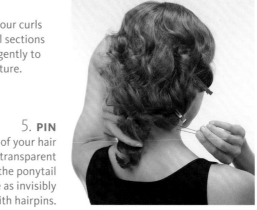

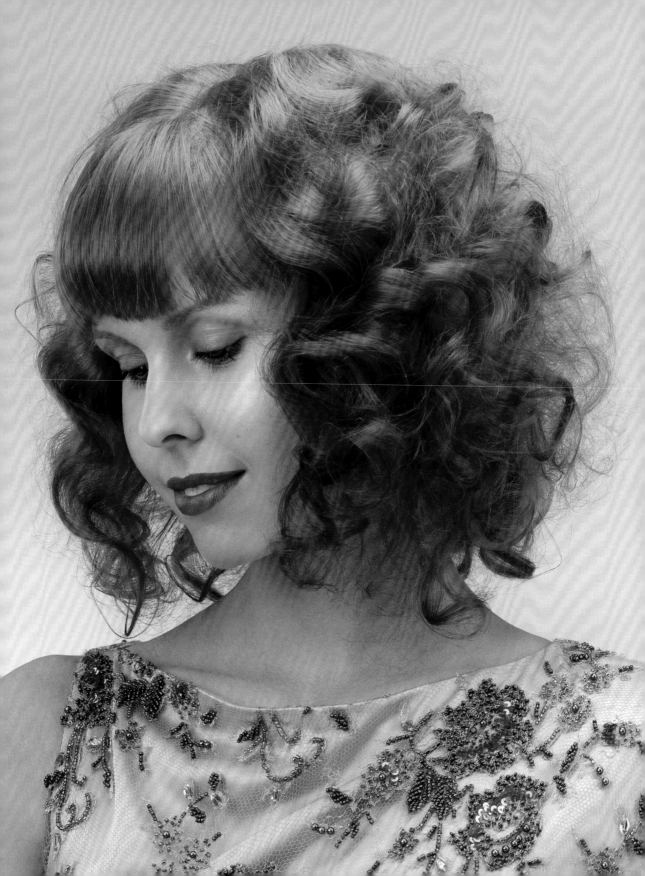

SOFT WAVES

Want "roaring twenties"-style soft waves? Here you go! This curling technique is suitable for completely straight hair or natural waves, and is quick and easy to do – no perming involved!

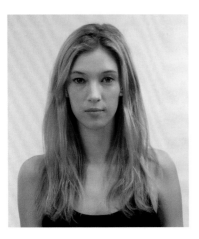

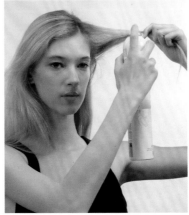

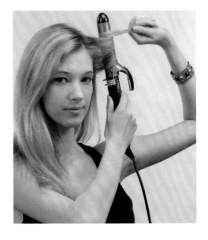

1. PART
These waves look especially luxurious and glamorous in over-shoulder-length hair. First, make a side parting – the style looks totally different with a centre parting.

2. PREPARE
Divide your hair into thin sections and spray it with hair lacquer. This has a setting effect, and will give your waves more elasticity and bounce.

3. WAVE
Wrap the sprayed strands around large-barrelled curling tongs. Then carefully remove the tongs, while holding the curl in place with your hand.

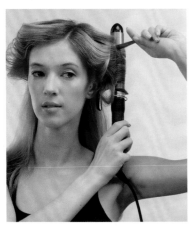

4. COOL
Pin each curl to your head with a hairgrip. Leave them to cool thoroughly, then remove the hairgrips, carefully brush out your hair, and tease it into shape with your fingers.

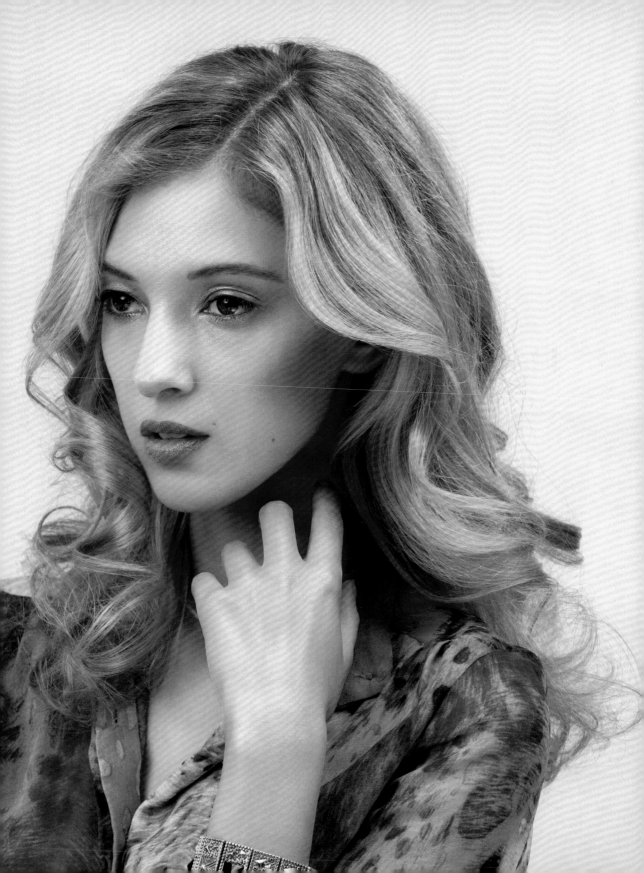

STRAIGHT HAIR

An elegant, sleek look is always on trend. With the right tricks and straightening methods, curls and waves – and even stubborn, frizzy hair – can be transformed into pure silk.

STRAIGHTENERS

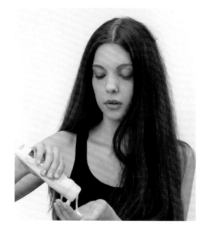

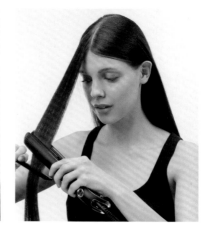

1. PROTECT
Very important: add a heat protection product to your hair before using heated tools. Straighteners can reach 220°C (430°F) , so your hair needs a fine protective coating.

2. DIVIDE
Brush most of your hair to one side and secure it with a large clip. Comb out a not-too-thin strand and put the straighteners around it, level with your temple.

3. STRAIGHTEN
Insert a comb just below the straighteners and comb your hair out as you go. Let the straighteners glide swiftly over your hair, without applying too much pressure.

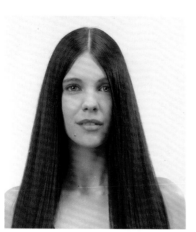

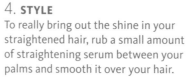

4. STYLE
To really bring out the shine in your straightened hair, rub a small amount of straightening serum between your palms and smooth it over your hair.

KERATIN STRAIGHTENING

If you don't want to straighten your hair every day, you can book a "discipline" treatment with your hairdresser, which will tame your hair for up to ten washes, without using chemicals. A morpho-keratin complex will give you beautifully straight hair from the inside out. This is how it works: an emulsion containing ceramides and amino acids is applied to damp hair, shaping it from within. Wheat proteins and positively charged polymers cling to the surface of the hair, combating frizz and adding shine from root to tip

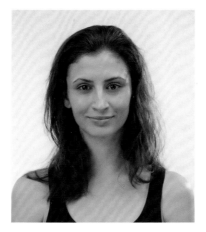

1. PREPARE
Before blow-drying with round brushes, shampoo and condition your hair as usual, brush well, and pre-blow-dry thoroughly to save time.

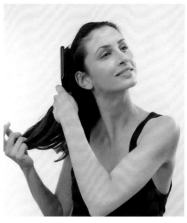

2. BRUSH IN
Add some blow-dry mousse to a brush, and brush it into your hair from root to tip. This will give your style hold, and protect your hair from heat and frizz.

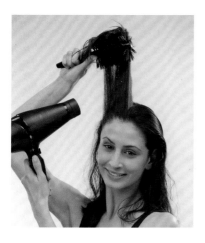

3. ROLL UP
Separate a strand and pull a large round brush through it several times, keeping some tension in your hair. Start blow-drying with the roots and work towards the ends.

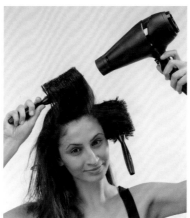

4. DRY
It's quicker to work with several round brushes, if you have them. Important: always leave the brush to cool in your hair for a while, to give the style more hold.

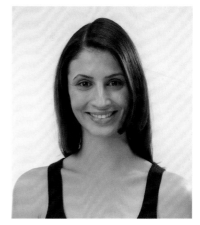

5. STYLE
Finally, brush out your straightened hair, shape it as desired and hold it in place with some shine hairspray.

SLEEK WET-LOOK

Your hair doesn't always need to be super shiny. This deliberately casual, just-got-out-of-bed look is very hip and gives long hair a structured but wild look.

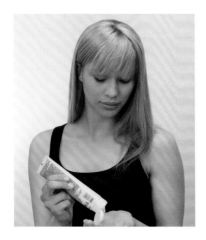 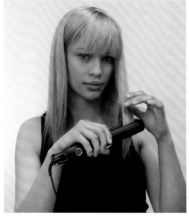 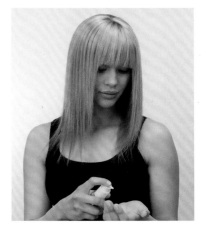

1. PROTECT
Make a centre parting, comb your hair straight and apply a heat protection product (gel or spray) all over it. Pay particular attention to the sensitive tips.

2. STRAIGHTEN
Straighten your hair, sliding the straighteners lightly over thin sections. Keep the straighteners at the same angle all the way to the tips for perfectly straight hair.

3. COMB
Finally, straighten your fringe and carefully comb your hair out. Squeeze a little styling serum into your hand.

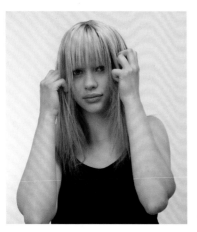

4. STYLE
Rub the serum between your palms and work it into your hair, from ear level down. Caution: don't add any product to your roots as it will make your hair look greasy.

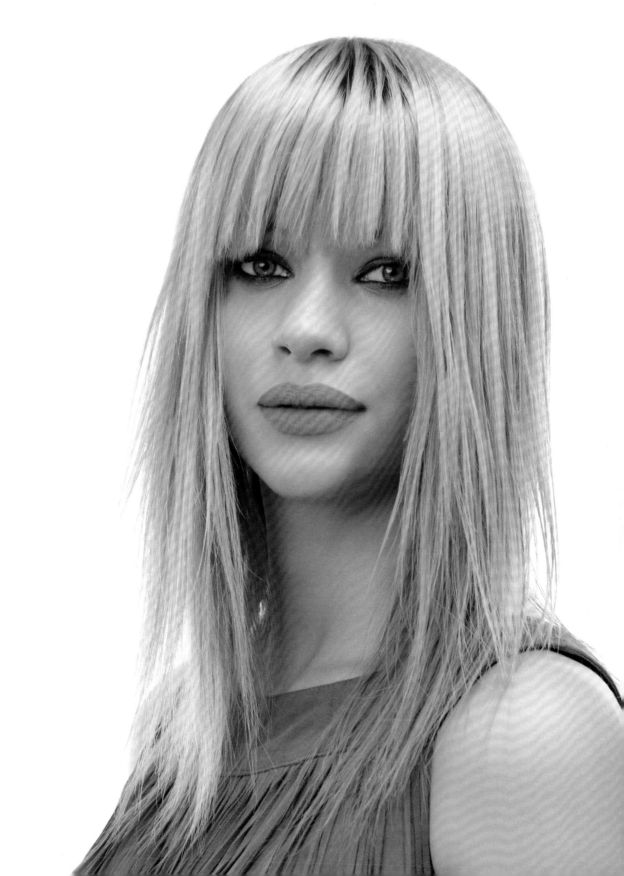

MID-LENGTH STYLE

This long bob is also known as a clavicut. Clavicle is another word for collarbone, and that's exactly where your hair will end. This length flatters your face, while your hair is still long enough to be styled into a ponytail or updo.

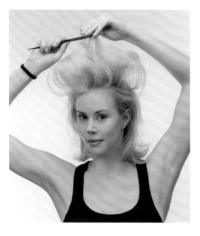

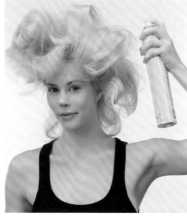

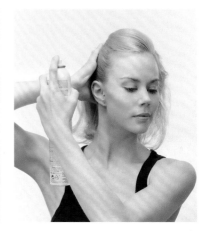

1. BACKCOMB
First brush your hair well, then thoroughly back comb the hair on the top of your head. Thin, fine hair may need a bit of structural spray as well.

2. SPRAY
Backcomb the sides and back with a steel comb as well. Add some hairspray as you go to give your hair more grip and a longer hold.

3. SMOOTH
Brush the surface of your hair and clip the side sections behind your ears. Use a lot of hairspray and the flat of your hand to smooth them down, and let the spray dry.

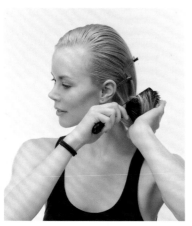

4. SHAPE
Use a hairdryer and brush to flick the ends of your hair outwards. Carefully remove the clips and brush the style through gently, or just shape with your hands.

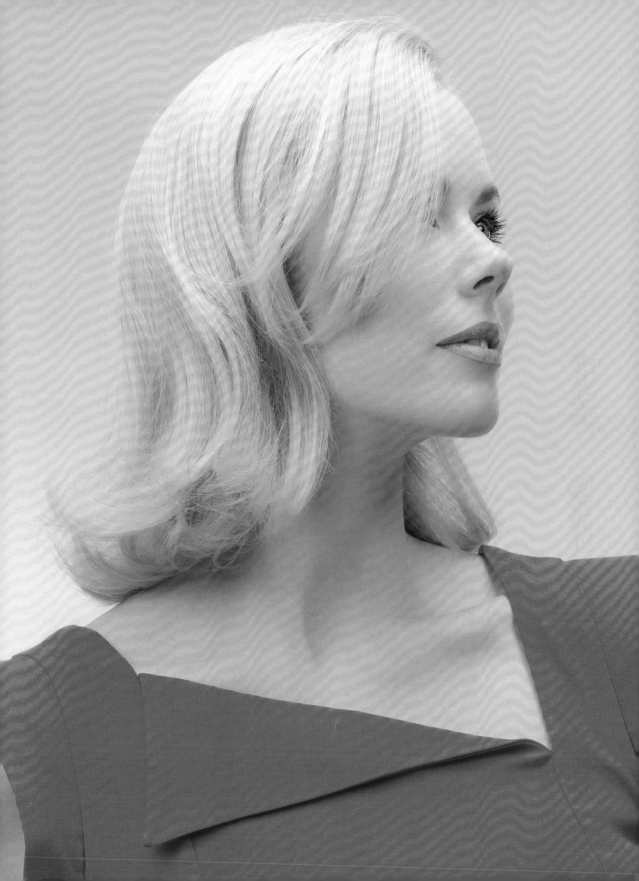

1 CUT – 4 LOOKS
A VERSATILE BOB

There are many advantages to having a bob: it suits women of all ages, works with straight or slightly wavy hair, and even makes much more of thin or fine hair. Boring? Definitely not if you know how many ways there are to style it...

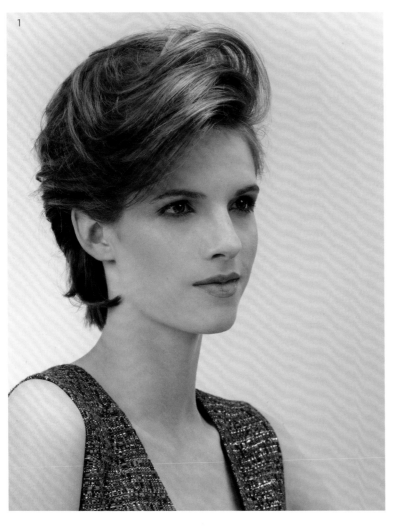

1

1. SOPHISTICATED

This variation, with a lavish quiff, looks elegant, but is far from prim. Work some styling mousse into towel-dried hair and brush it through from roots to tips. Pre-blow-dry well, and then blow-dry your hair in sections with a medium-sized round brush. Important: for long-lasting volume, always leave the round brush in your hair for a while to cool after blow-drying. Using several round brushes speeds the process up. Finally, brush through and style to one side. A bit of backcombing and a lot of hairspray will give you even more volume.

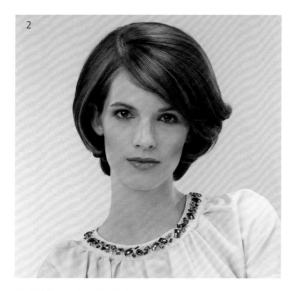

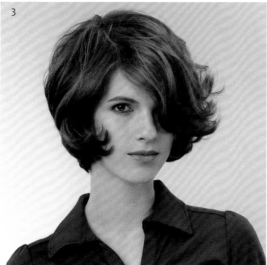

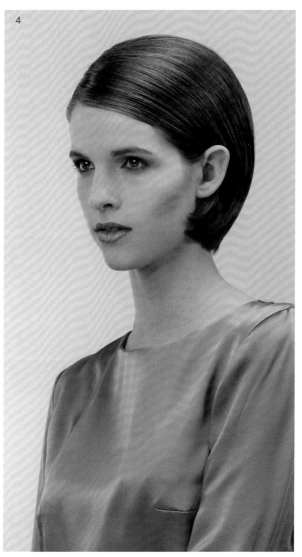

2. CLASSIC

Rounded and pretty, blow dried to give you lots of volume, this is an office-friendly bob. To style: work some setting mousse into damp hair and pre-blow-dry thoroughly. Blow-dry in sections over a large round brush, so that your hair turns under slightly. Bring the side fringe down over your forehead and use hairspray to give the whole look more hold.

3. PLAYFUL

A bit of a wave will give your bob a soft, feminine look. Work styling mousse into damp hair and blow-dry with medium-sized round brushes, or Velcro/heated rollers. Leave your hair to cool before removing the rollers. Brush out, and tease into shape with fingers and a little styling creme. Fix with hairspray.

4. TRENDY

This bob looks sleek and narrow. Use straighteners to straighten your hair in sections, turning the ends under slightly as you go. Brush through, then rub a little styling creme between your palms and smooth it over your hair. A spritz of shine spray will keep it looking glamorous.

SIDE CHIGNON

Very sophisticated, very classic – but with a cheeky edge: the difference in this asymmetric chignon lies in the low side-parting and the strands falling low over the forehead.

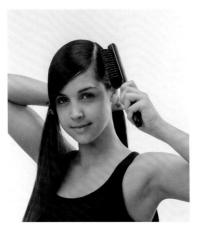

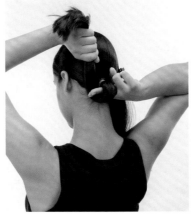

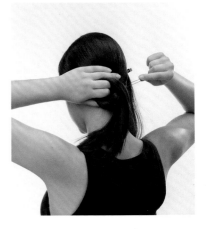

1. BRUSH
Give yourself a low side-parting. Separate a wide section of hair above your right ear and pin it to one side. Tie the rest of your hair back into an off-centre ponytail.

2. LOOP
Put two fingers under your ponytail and wrap it around them, not too tightly, to form a loop. Then remove your fingers and hold the chignon in place.

3. PIN
Pin the loop in place invisibly using several hairpins. Then unpin the section above your ear, back-comb it, and smooth the surface back down with a styling brush.

THE DAY AFTER
Hair can be soft and slippery just after it's been washed. For an updo, however, it needs a bit of grip and volume. Setting mousse, structure spray, or salt spray will make your hair easier to shape and style. If you can, wash your hair the night before for easier styling.

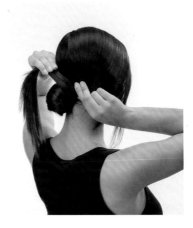

4. CONCEAL
Wrap the loose section round the chignon several times, like a hairband made of your own hair. Fix securely in place with hairpins. Tease out a thin strand at the front.

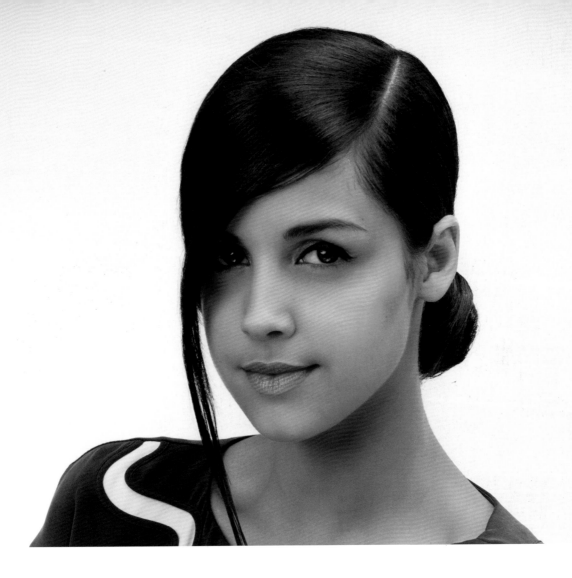

*Variation:
bringing your
hair down over
your forehead like
a side fringe makes
for an even more
elegant look.*

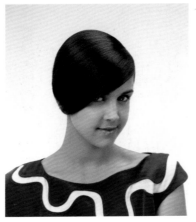

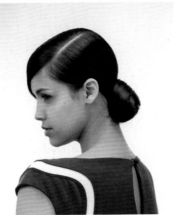

BASIC TECHNIQUES
THE PONYTAIL

It helps us deal with bad hair days; it's probably the quickest style for long hair, and it ranges from classy to trendy. You'll be surprised at how many options there are...

FROM SIMPLE TO STATEMENT

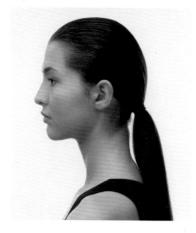

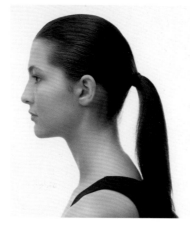

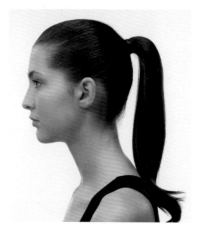

1. SOPHISTICATED
Worn low on the neck, this ponytail looks very elegant, and goes perfectly with simple outfits for an understated look.

2. CLASSIC
The all-rounder that goes with everything, from a blazer and chinos for the office, to joggers and vest for the gym. It should sit at about ear height.

3. SPORTY
Swept straight back, this ponytail looks confident and self-assured. Make a sporty fashion statement, or wear it to the gym.

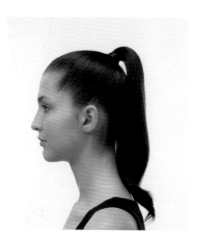

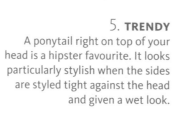

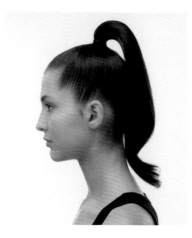

4. PLAYFUL
A ponytail sitting very high on the back of your head makes for a sensational profile, adding volume to the top section of your hair. Makes rounded faces appear narrower.

5. TRENDY
A ponytail right on top of your head is a hipster favourite. It looks particularly stylish when the sides are styled tight against the head and given a wet look.

SOFTLY DOES IT

If you wear a ponytail a lot, you should really use a high-quality hairband. Transparent mini hairbands are nice and stretchy, but they are only meant to be used once. They wear out quickly and can become brittle. Bands that have a metal staple in them can damage hair, and aren't suitable for constant use. Ideally, you want a fabric-covered hairband without a join. It should be as stretchy as possible, so that it doesn't rip out too many hairs when you take your ponytail out.

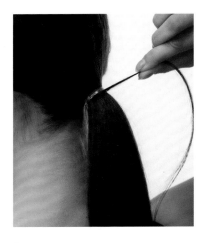

1. TIE

Once you have tied your ponytail with a transparent hairband, take a very thin strand of hair from underneath and wrap it two or three times around the hairband.

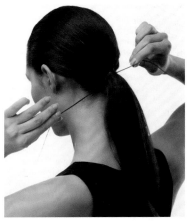

2. COVER

Take a second thin strand from under your ponytail and wrap it in the same direction as the first, until the hairband is completely covered.

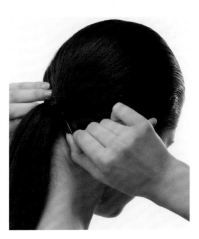

3. FIX

Pin the ends of the two wrapped strands in place underneath the ponytail, as invisibly as possible. Use hairpins that match your hair colour.

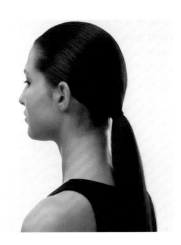

4. STYLE

The fine ends of the two strands should finish behind the hairband. Hold the style in place with extra-strong hairspray.

SIXTIES FOUNTAIN

A bit retro, but still trendy: this updo is something very special. Styling takes a bit of time, but the results are really worth it.

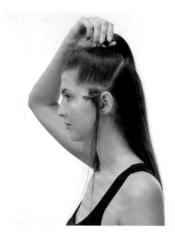

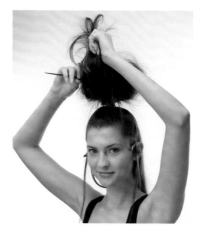

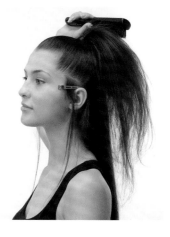

1. DIVIDE
Separate a thin strand just above each ear and fix with a clip. Bring together about a third of the hair from the top of your head, and tie it tightly with a hairband.

2. CREATE VOLUME
Backcomb the ponytail on top of your head thoroughly with a steel comb. Use a little structure spray as you go for even more volume and grip.

3. SMOOTH
Use a shallow brush to smooth down the surface of the backcombed section, being careful not to lose any of the volume you've created.

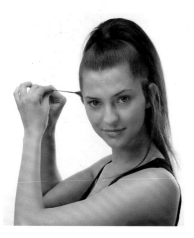

4. TWIST
Twist the two strands above your ears with your fingertips, then lay them around the back of your head and over the fountain ponytail. Pin each in place behind the opposite ear.

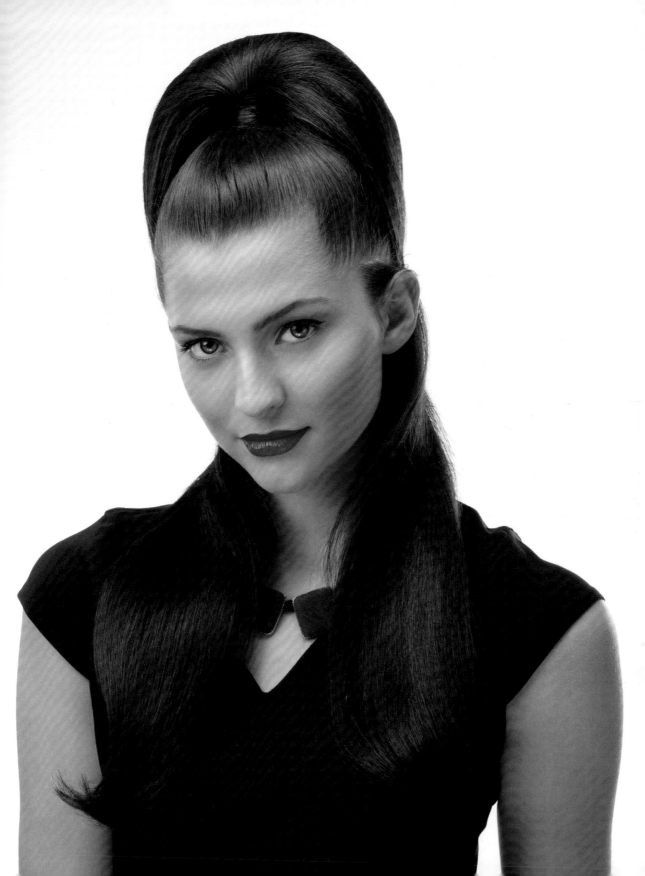

ROLLOVER PONYTAIL

What would you say to a more refined version of a ponytail that's still super quick to style? A little twist, a double roll, and there you go: a ponytail that will ensure all eyes are on you.

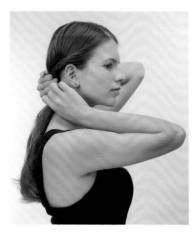

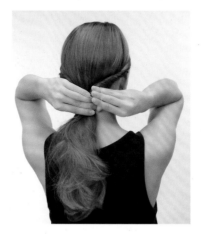

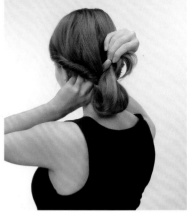

1. **TWIST**
Make a side parting and brush your hair smooth. Starting at your temple on either side, twist a not-too-thin strand, and pull it back along with the rest of your hair.

2. **TIE**
Tie the two twisted strands and the rest of your hair together into a low ponytail, using a transparent hairband.

3. **PULL THROUGH**
Put one finger through the ponytail from underneath, between the hairband and your head, and pull the end of the ponytail all the way through to make it shorter.

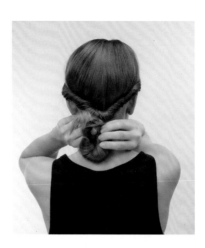

4. **ROLL OVER**
For longer than shoulder-length hair, repeat the rollover move. If your hair is shoulder length or shorter, once will be enough.

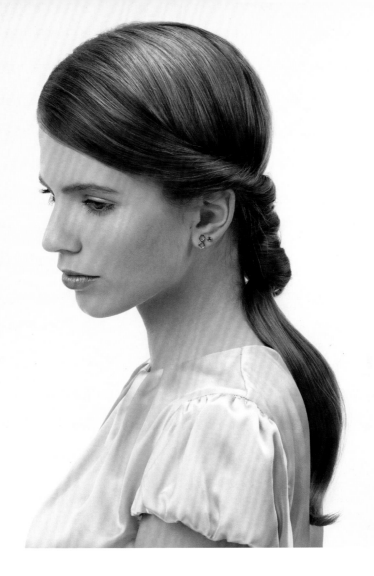

Variation: after pulling through, divide the ponytail in two, then twist and tie in three places.

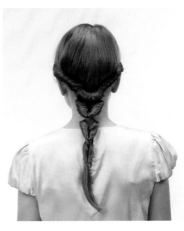

FAKING IT

Want truly big hair for once? The best way is to use a hairpiece. High quality hairpieces are almost impossible to tell from real hair in colour and structure, and provide striking effects.

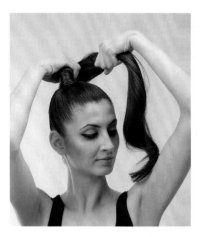

1. TWIST
Tie your hair into a ponytail on top of your head with a hairband. Turn the ponytail around itself several times, wrapping it into a high bun.

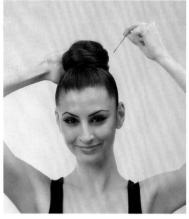

2. PIN
Pin the bun securely into place with hairpins. Make sure the knot is really high on the top of your head, or the hairpiece won't hold properly.

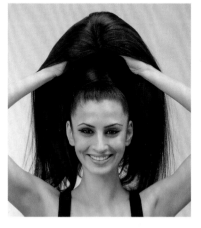

3. PLACE
Take hold of the hairpiece from inside and place it on top of the chignon like a hat. If your bun doesn't create enough volume, use a hair pad.

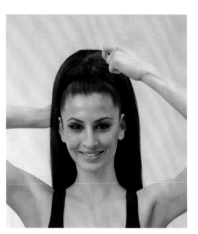

4. ARRANGE
Fix the hairpiece to your own hair very securely with hairpins so that it doesn't slip. A little extra-strong hairspray will give you a secure hold.

ALL HAIR IS NOT EQUAL
Hairpieces and wigs come in various qualities. The differences lie in the material that the hair is fixed onto, the way the hair is attached, and the hair quality (whether artificial hair or real hair from Asia or Europe). A high-quality piece is up to 100 per cent hand-knotted, using mostly European hair.

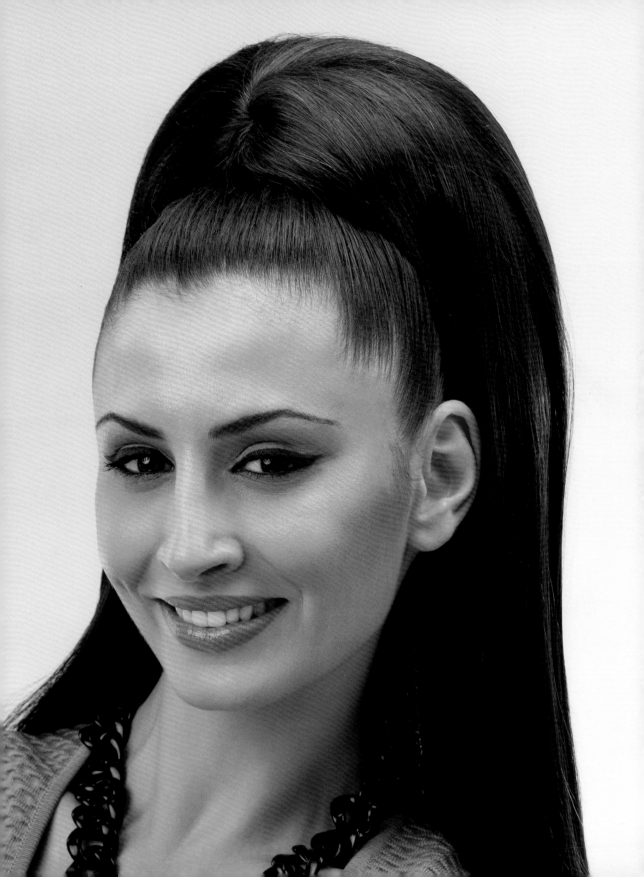

MESSY PONYTAIL

Want hair that looks as natural as possible? This is a style that doesn't look styled: a soft, windswept ponytail, with gentle volume that will flatter your face.

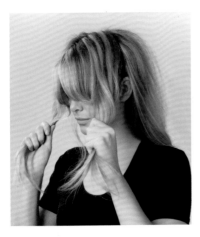

1. DIVIDE
Make a horizontal parting from one ear to the other, and separate out a thick section on either side. Twist each into a coil and hold it in place with hair clips.

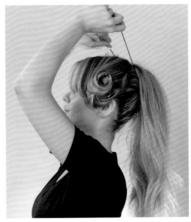

2. LIFT
Backcomb the roots of the rest of your hair and pull it into a high ponytail using an open-ended, stretchy rubber band.

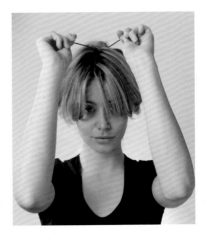

3. TIE
Knot the rubber band and pull it tight. Take the clips out of the side sections and let the loose hair fall forward.

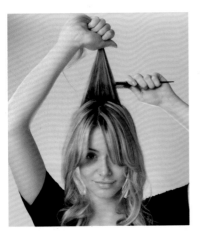

4. BACKCOMB
Backcomb the top section thoroughly, then bring it back over the ponytail and tie it up with the rubber band as well, knotting the band again.

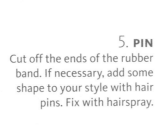

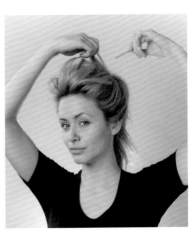

5. PIN
Cut off the ends of the rubber band. If necessary, add some shape to your style with hair pins. Fix with hairspray.

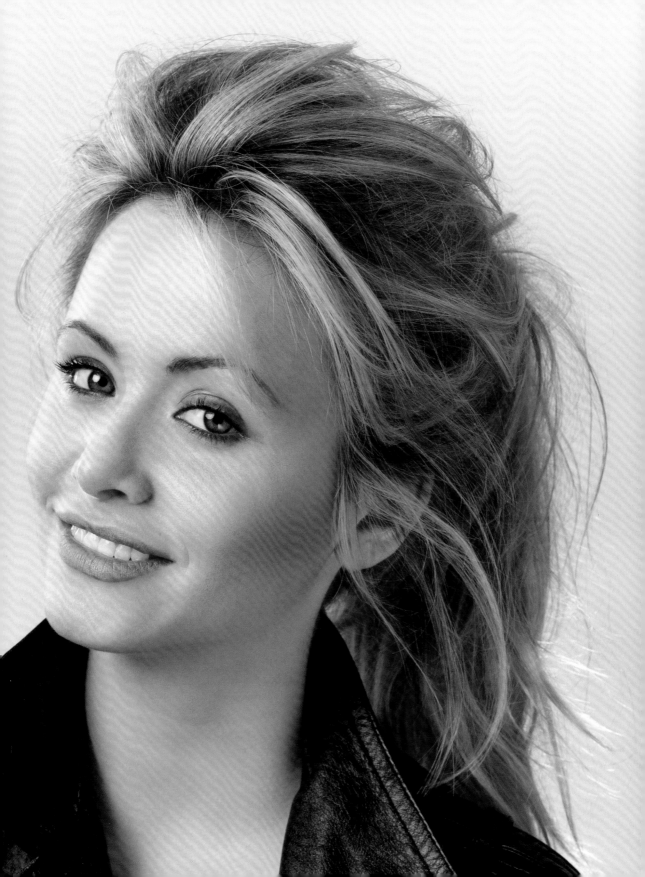

BASIC TECHNIQUES
BRAIDING TECHNIQUES

An artistic braid always looks good, and has the potential to become a classic. Way too complicated? Not necessarily. Master a few basic variations, and you can whip up a great effect in no time.

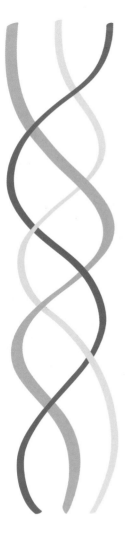

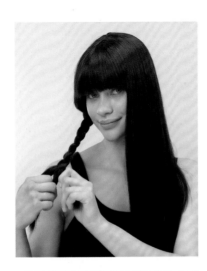

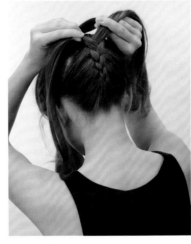

1. **FRENCH AND DUTCH BRAIDS**
Both braids are usually done using three strands, but there are also more difficult variations that use five. For a French braid (top picture), which is sometimes called an invisible braid, the strands are laid over each other. For a Dutch braid (lower picture) or reverse French braid, the strands are placed under one another. For the basic three-strand variation, separate out a section of hair on the top of your head and divide it into three strands. If you're doing a French braid, lay the right-hand strand over the middle one, and for a Dutch braid lay it underneath. Then lay the left-hand strand over (French) or under (Dutch) the middle one. The left-hand strand will now be in the middle. Then add a little more hair from the right-hand side of your head to the right-hand strand, and bring this into the middle as before. Add a little more hair to the left-hand strand and bring it into the middle. Carry on until you have added all your hair into the braid.

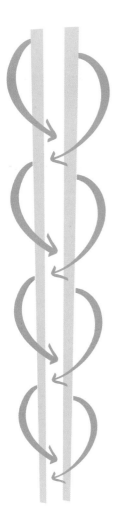

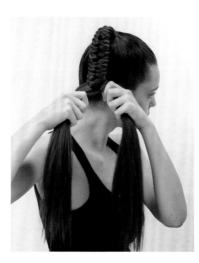

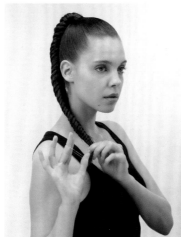

2. FISHTAIL BRAID

The fishtail is an on-trend braid with an interesting structure. Braided tightly, the pattern looks classic; braided loosely it looks cool and casual. This is how the herringbone braid works: separate a section at the top of your head and divide it into two large strands using the index finger of your right hand. Now take a thin strand from the outside of the let-hand section and add it to the inside of the right-hand section. Then change hands, and hold the sections apart with the index finger of your left hand. Take a thin strand from the outside of the right-hand section and add it to the inside of the left-hand section. Then change hands again and repeat the process. Important: make sure the strands you are braiding in, and the two main sections, are always the same thickness, to give you a regular pattern. Carry on like this until all the hair is braided.

EASY BRAIDS

Bring out your inner Native American: the primary school classic is back, and it looks cute on grown women too, especially worn in combination with a full fringe.

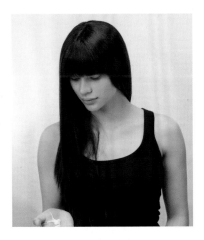

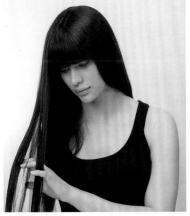

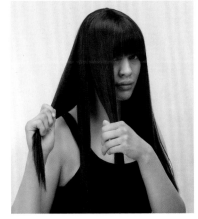

1. PREPARE
Make a centre parting and brush your hair completely smooth with a paddle brush. Take a small amount of styling cream and rub it into the palm of your hand.

2. WORK IN
Comb your fingers through your hair, working the styling cream into it. This will ensure your hair stays shiny, and no frizz escapes from the braids.

3. SEPARATE
Comb your hair once more and make a straight centre parting all the way down to the back of your neck. Divide the hair on either side into three equal-sized strands.

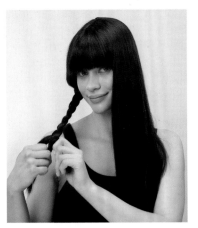

4. BRAID
Braid the three strands on one side together into quite a tight braid, and tie off the end with a transparent hairband. Then do the same with the other side.

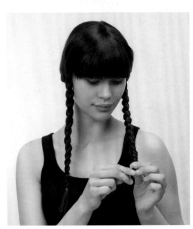

5. FIX
Tie off the second braid with a hairband. Finally, loosen individual loops of hair with your fingers to give the braids more body.

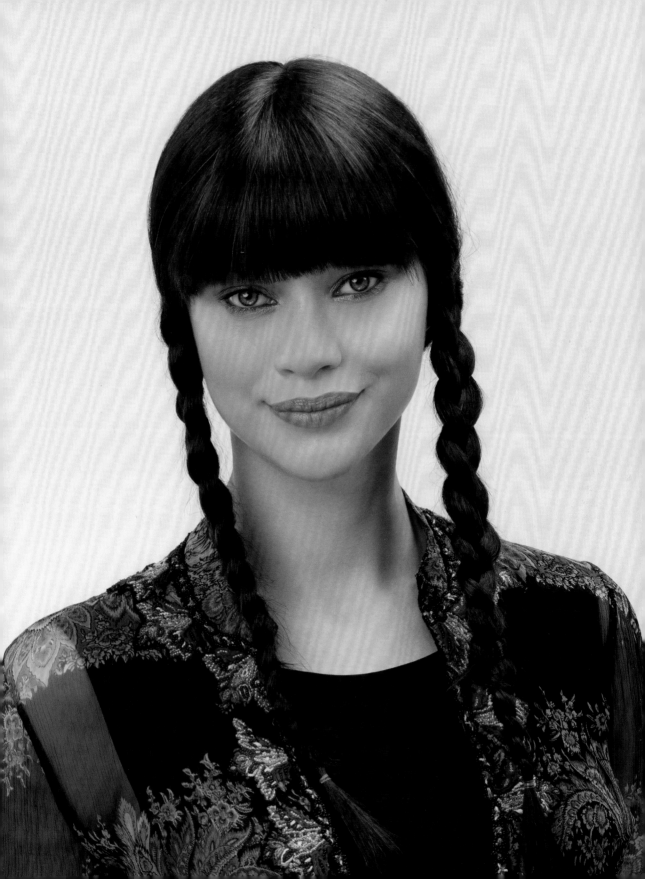

MODERN HEIDI

Braided styles never go out of fashion. This crown braid is inspired by a German folk style, and has a romantic look. Thick hair will produce a particularly good sculpted effect.

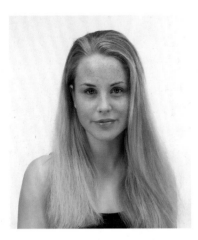

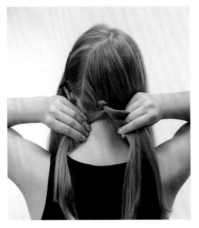

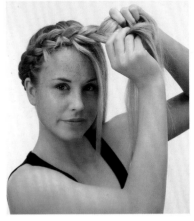

1. PREPARE
For a crown braid, hair should ideally be well over shoulder-length. First, make a side parting and brush out your hair thoroughly.

2. DIVIDE
Take a central section at the nape of your neck. Divide it into three, take the strands in both hands and braid the right strand, then the l eft, over the middle strand.

3. BRAID
Take some hair from the right and add it into the right strand, then braid this strand into the middle. Take hair from the left into the left strand and braid it into the middle.

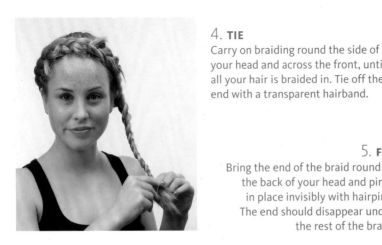

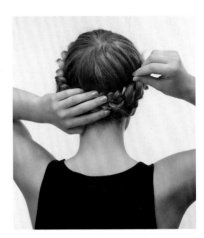

4. TIE
Carry on braiding round the side of your head and across the front, until all your hair is braided in. Tie off the end with a transparent hairband.

5. FIX
Bring the end of the braid round to the back of your head and pin it in place invisibly with hairpins. The end should disappear under the rest of the braid.

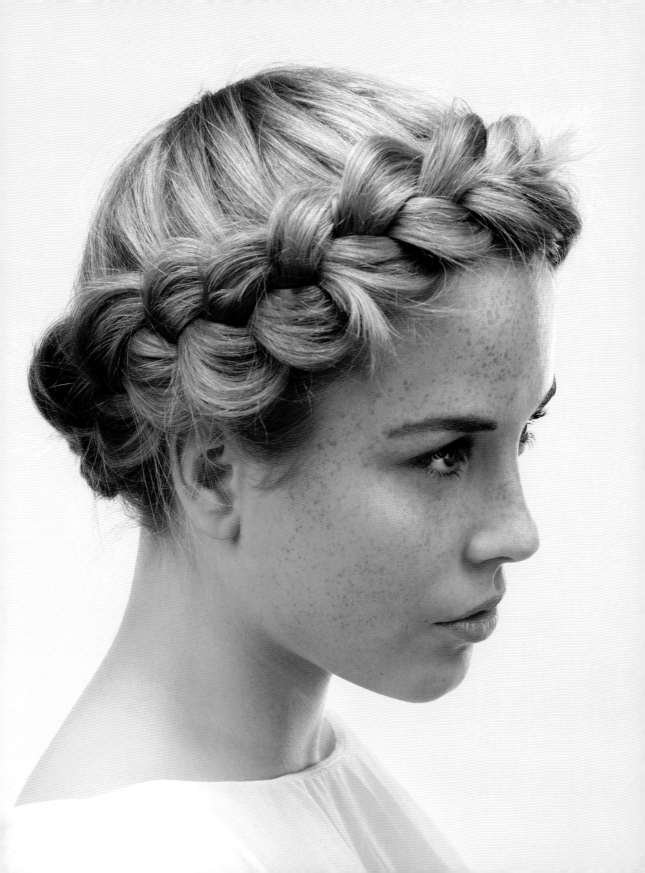

HIGH HERRINGBONE BRAID

The herringbone braid's three-dimensional structure gives it an artistic edge, and, depending on how you style it, can look either romantic or fashionable. Don't worry: the technique is much less complicated than the results make it look.

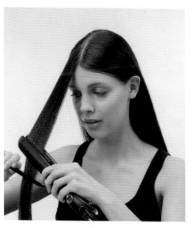

1. STRAIGHTEN
Make a centre parting, brush your hair and straighten it section by section, using a light pressure and pulling a comb through below the straighteners as you go.

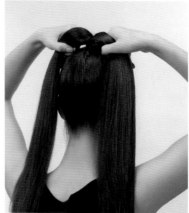

2. TIE
Tie your hair up into a very high ponytail with a hairband, and separate it into two equal sections. Spray in a little structure spray for better hold.

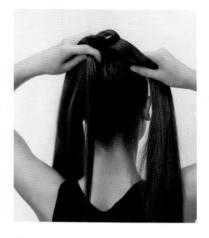

3. DIVIDE
Take a thin strand from the outside of the left section and add it to the inside of the right section. Then take a strand from the outside right and add it to the inside left.

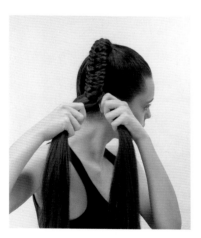

4. BRAID
Carry on until all your hair is braided. Make sure both sections stay the same thickness, so that the result looks regular.

5. TIE
Tie off the bottom of the finished fishtail with a clear hairband. You can also add a decorative hair band to the top of the braid.

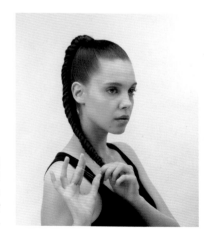

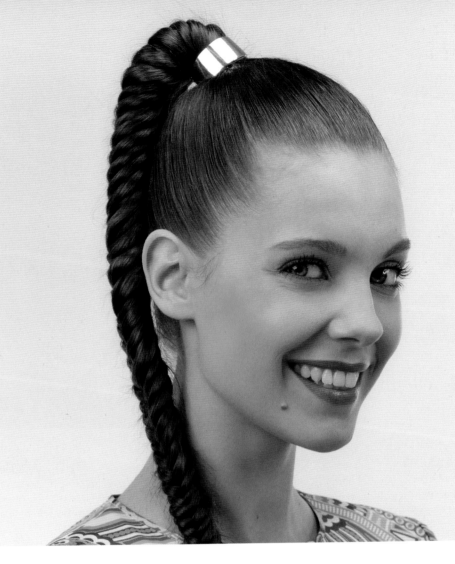

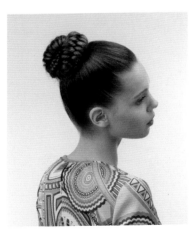

*Variation:
coiled and pinned,
the fishtail braid
becomes an instant
structured chignon.*

BRAIDED CHIGNON

A romantic braided look, with a French braid and an offset chignon providing the star attraction. A great summer festival look that also works for the office, or as a glamorous evening updo.

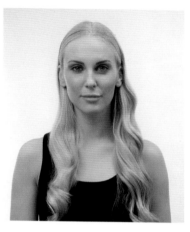

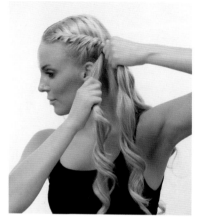

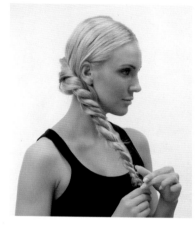

1. PART
For this style your hair should be well over shoulder length, or the chignon won't work. Brush your hair out and part it wherever you like.

2. BRAID
Separate out three strands from the top front section, on the side with more hair. Braid the right then the left strand over the middle one, twisting each as you go.

3. PUT UP
Take some hair to the right of the braid and add to the right strand, then braid it into the middle. Take hair to the left of the braid and add it to the left strand.

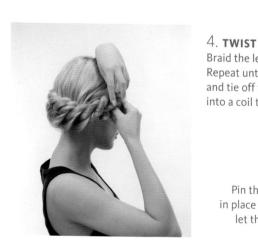

4. TWIST
Braid the left strand into the middle. Repeat until all your hair is braided, and tie off the end. Twist your hair into a coil that sits low on your neck.

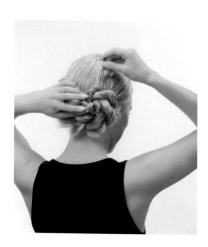

5. FIX
Pin the braided chignon securely in place with hairpins, trying not to let the pins show. Fix with some extra-strong hairspray.

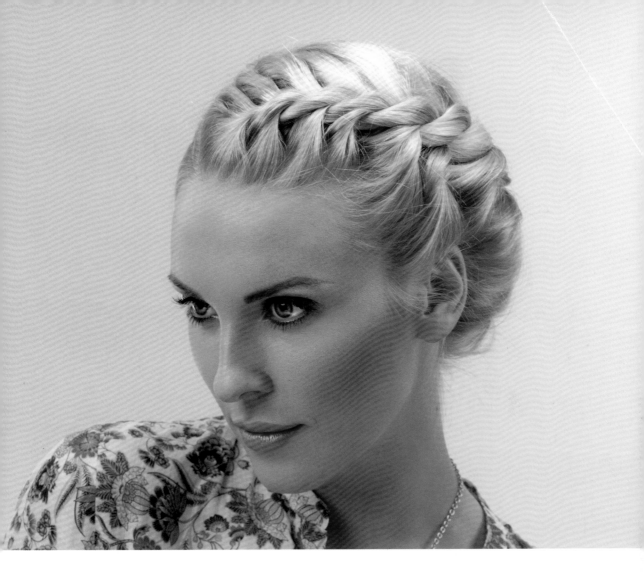

A bit Heidi, a bit ballerina: this updo looks different from every angle.

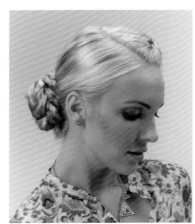
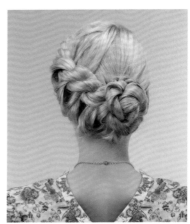

CASUAL CURLY BRAID

Less ornamental, but with an appeal all of its own: the little hairline braid detail is what makes this look special. Perfect for shoulder-length hair – and natural waves are welcome!

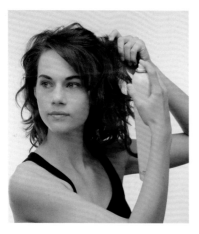

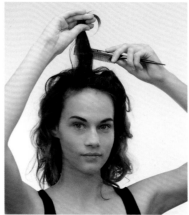

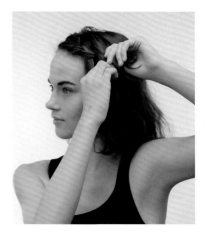

1. **ADD BODY**
To make wavy hair look even more casual, spray some hairspray onto it from underneath. This will give you loads of volume, and make your waves look more structured.

2. **CREATE SOME GRIP**
Backcomb the front section thoroughly with a steel comb to give your braid a more luxurious look. Gently comb the surface of the hair back down.

3. **BRAID**
Starting at your side parting and working towards the opposite ear, give yourself a French braid (instructions on p.76). Work loosely for a softer appearance.

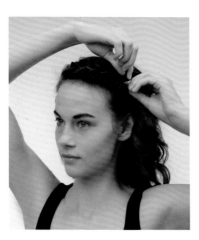

4. **PIN**
Fix the braid in place at ear height, using a hairgrip or a decorated clip. The end will fall softly into the rest of your hair.

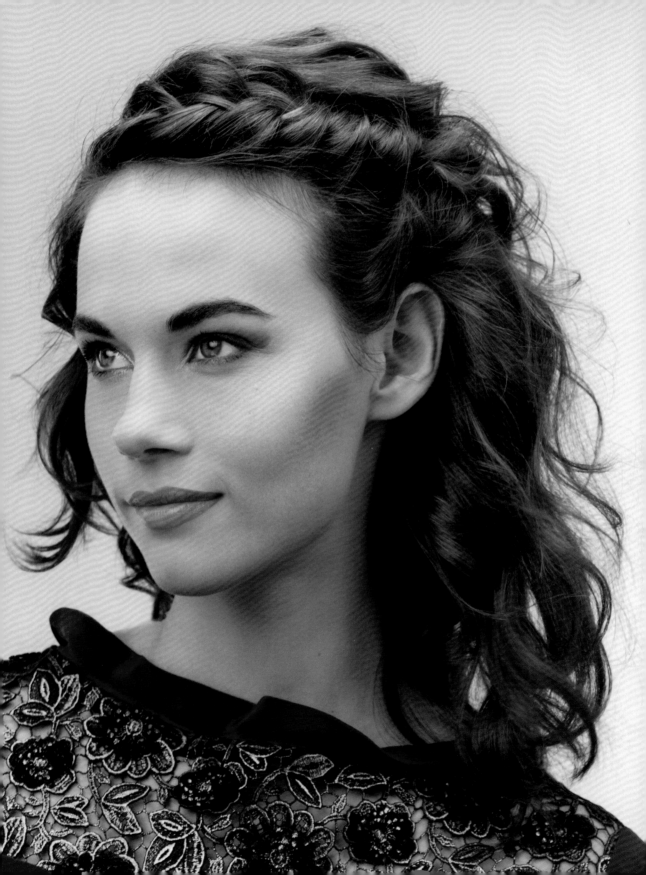

DIRECTIONAL DUTCH BRAID

The Dutch braid is a classic, and the structure looks particularly good in relatively thick hair. But with a little backcombing, even women with fine hair can do a lot more with less.

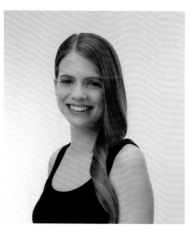

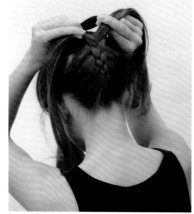

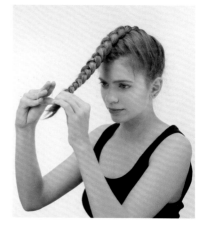

1. PREPARE
For a Dutch braid your hair should be at least shoulder-length. Work a little extra-strong hairspray into your hair for more grip.

2. BRAID
Starting at the nape of your neck, separate three strands. Braid the right strand, then the left under the middle strand. Gather a little more hair into the right strand.

3. PICK UP
Braid the right strand under the middle one again, then take a little hair from the left side into the left strand. Carry on until all your hair is braided.

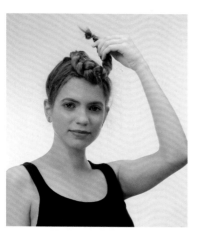

4. COIL
Tie off the end with a hair band, and twist the braid into a coil at the front of your head. Hide the end of the braid under the coil.

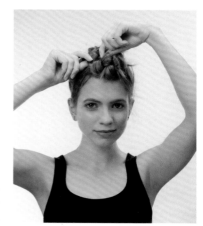

5. PIN
Fix your work of art in place securely with hairpins. Add some extra-strong hairspray for extra hold.

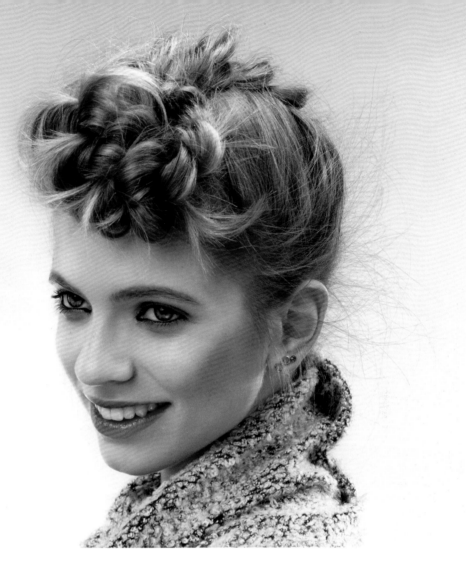

Beautiful hair, however you look at it: from the front, back or in profile.

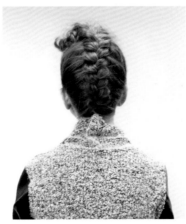 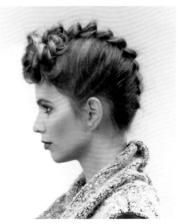

89

BRAID-PATTERNED CHIGNON

A style best suited to very long, thick hair, which will emphasize the sculpted effect of this simple braid. However, even with fine hair, the braid turns this chignon into a real feature.

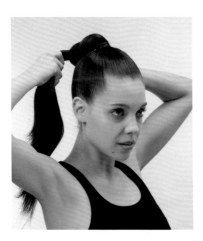

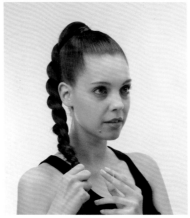

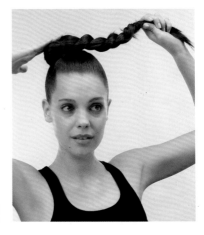

1. **BRAID**
Brush your hair smooth and tie it into a high ponytail with a hairband. Separate the ponytail into two equal strands, twist them and wrap them around each other.

2. **FIX**
Keep hold of the strands to make sure they stay twisted. Finally, tie off the end of the braid with a transparent hairband.

3. **COIL**
Twist the braid into a coil that sits tight against your head. Hold the chignon down with one hand while you coil the braid around itself with the other.

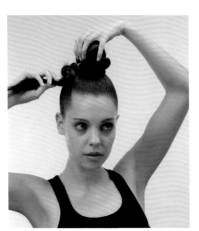

4. **CONCEAL**
Hide the end of the braid under the chignon. Tip: work with both hands until you're completely finished, so that no hair escapes or unravels.

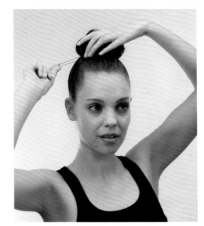

5. **SECURE**
Finally, secure the chignon invisibly with hairpins. A good coating of hairspray will make sure this glamorous look holds for hours.

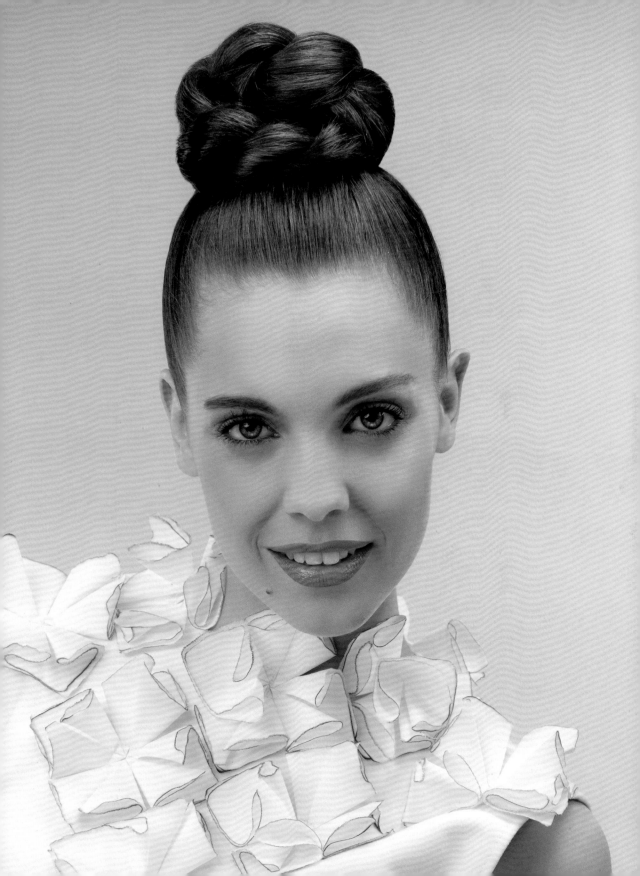

BASIC TECHNIQUES
THE CHIGNON

You could call it a bun, but chignon sounds more elegant. Either way, this is an updo inspired by ballerinas. The chignon can be styled with precision and glamour, or made to look soft and casual.

CLASSIC HIGH CHIGNON

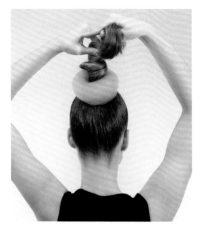

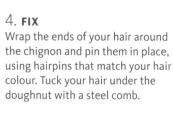

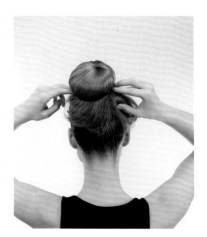

1. PUT ON
Tie all your hair neatly into a ponytail and pull it through a hair doughnut. Twist your hair until the majority of it has disappeared inside the pad.

2. ARRANGE
Spread the rest of your hair equally over the doughnut until it is completely covered, with a hole in the middle. Stretch a large hairband between your fingers.

3. TIE
Carefully bring the hairband down over the doughnut until it is sitting below it, at the root of the ponytail. The ends of your hair will still stick out around the band.

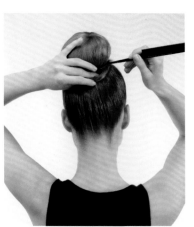

4. FIX
Wrap the ends of your hair around the chignon and pin them in place, using hairpins that match your hair colour. Tuck your hair under the doughnut with a steel comb.

5. STYLE
Fix your extra-large bun in place with lots of extra-strong hairspray, and give the sides of your hair a gleaming wet look.

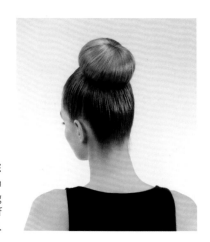

QUICK CHANGE ARTIST

An asymmetrically placed chignon can be a really interesting look. You can wear a side bun either low on your neck, or high up on your head. For a casual, "just back from the beach" updo, put your head down, brush all your hair forwards, twist it into a knot high on your head and fix it in place with a transparent hairband. Tease out a few strands and let them fall over your face, to make it look as if your hair has been tousled by a sea breeze.

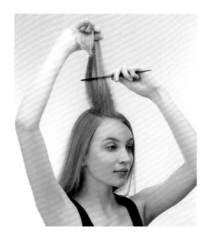

1. BACKCOMB

Backcomb your roots all the way round to stop your hair from separating. Structure spray will give you more hold. Smooth down the surface with a hairbrush.

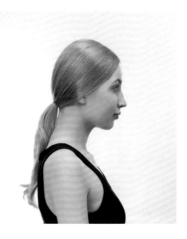

2. TIE

Brush your hair back and tie it into quite a loose, low ponytail. Your hair should cover your ears.

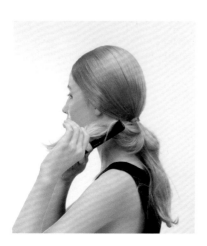

3. CREATE VOLUME

Separate your ponytail into two or three strands, add more structure spray, and backcomb it thoroughly.

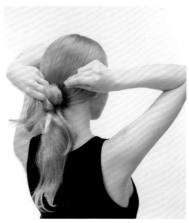

4. TWIST

Take each strand in turn and twist it around itself into a loose coil, before pinning it to the base of the ponytail with hairpins, as invisibly as possible.

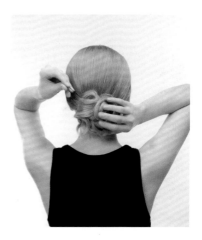

5. SHAPE

Shape the loose bun with your hands, and secure it with more hairpins. Some extra-strong hairspray will give you longer hold and shine.

UPDO WITH QUIFF

With a rock 'n' roll quiff for a rebellious edge, a traditional braid, and a French roll for a pinch of elegance, this unusual updo is literally multifaceted, making it perfect for all kinds of occasions.

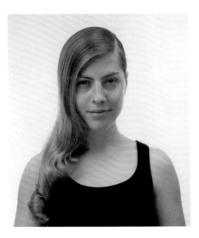

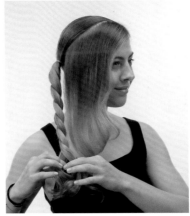

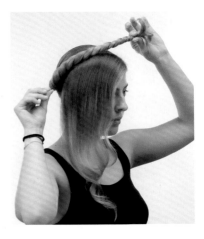

1. PREPARE
Your hair should be at least shoulder length. Make a low side parting from forehead to neck and tie your hair back at ear height, leaving a wide side section loose.

2. TWIST
Divide your ponytail in two and twist the strands together tightly, keeping it taut all the way down. Tie the end with a transparent hairband.

3. PLACE
Lay the braid along your diagonal parting and pin it there with hairpins. It will form a pad to create the volume for your quiff.

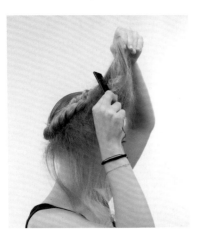

4. BACKCOMB
Backcomb the front side section thoroughly using a steel comb, and brush the surface smooth. You may want to use some structure spray.

5. PIN
Sweep the backcombed section back over the braid, tucking the ends of your hair underneath it at the back. Pin it in place with hairpins and fix with hairspray.

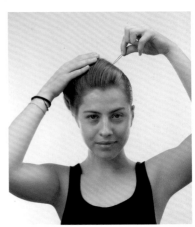

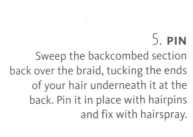

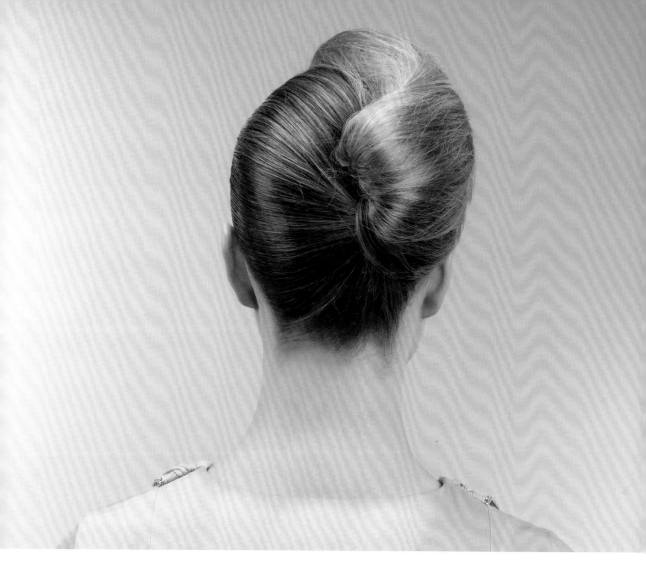

*One way or another:
a cool quiff up front;
elegant from the
side. And then there's
the back view...*

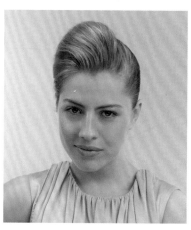

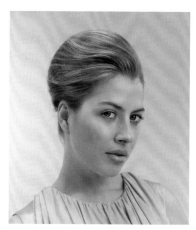

FAKE FRINGE UPDO

A fringe can be really flattering – but once you have one, you're stuck with it for a while. This style lets you see if a side fringe would suit you, with no obligations.

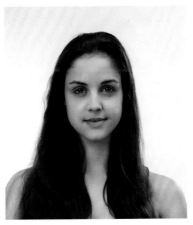

1. PREPARE
This look works particularly well on longer than shoulder length hair; your hair type is less important. Backcombing will give even fine hair sufficient body.

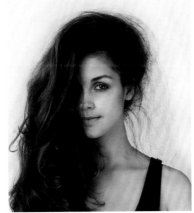

2. BACKCOMB
First, backcomb your hair to give it more grip and hold. You can increase hold even more by using a structure spray or extra-strong hairspray.

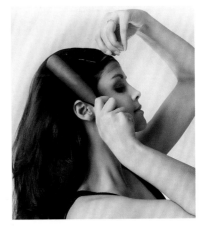

3. DIVIDE
Tilt your head back slightly and brush your hair to the side, pinning it in place with hairgrips as you wrap it around your head. Finally, sweep your hair across your forehead.

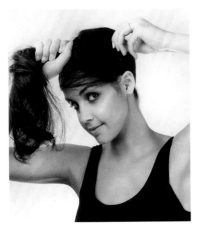

4. COVER
The backcombing shouldn't be visible, so brush the surface of your hair smooth. Some hair should fall over your forehead like a side fringe.

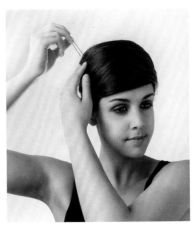

5. FIX
Merge the ends of your hair into the back of the updo, and pin them in place. Tease the fringe section further over your forehead. Fix everything with hairspray.

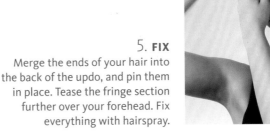

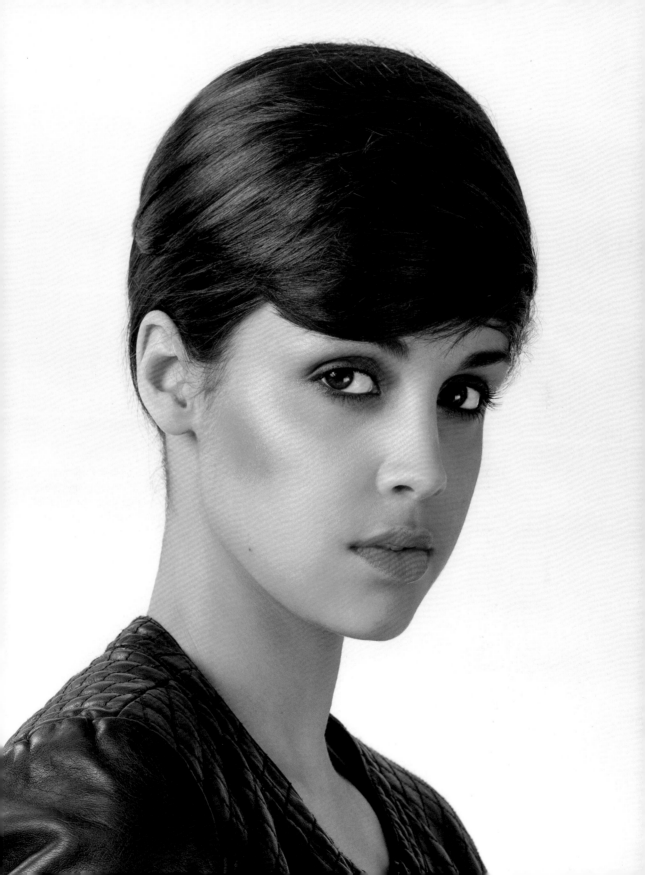

BEEHIVE

A beehive is a sophisticated but dressed-down look for straight or wavy hair longer than shoulder length. Do it like a pro and use a hair pad to create volume on top, giving loads more body to thin or fine hair.

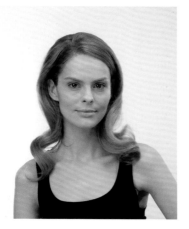

1. ARRANGE
Make a side parting and brush your hair into shape. If you have very fine, thin hair, add some mineral powder spray or volume powder to the roots and body.

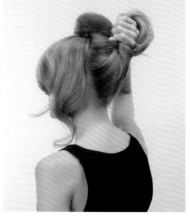

2. BRING TOGETHER
Divide your hair into three: one section on either side, and one at the back. Pin a hair pad to the top of your head and take hold of the back section in one hand.

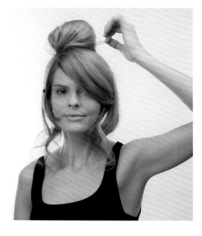

3. CONCEAL
Wrap this section of hair around the pad, covering it completely, and fix it securely in place with hairpins. You can also add a spritz of hairspray.

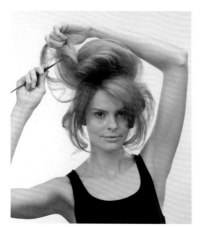

4. BACKCOMB
Separate the side sections into several strands and backcomb each one thoroughly. Then run a styling brush very lightly over the surface to smooth it down.

5. PIN
Use hairpins to pin the backcombed side sections up into a French roll below the pad at the back of your head. For a more casual look, tease out a few strands from the sides.

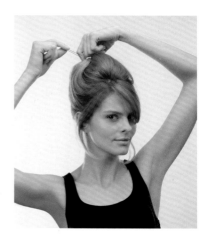

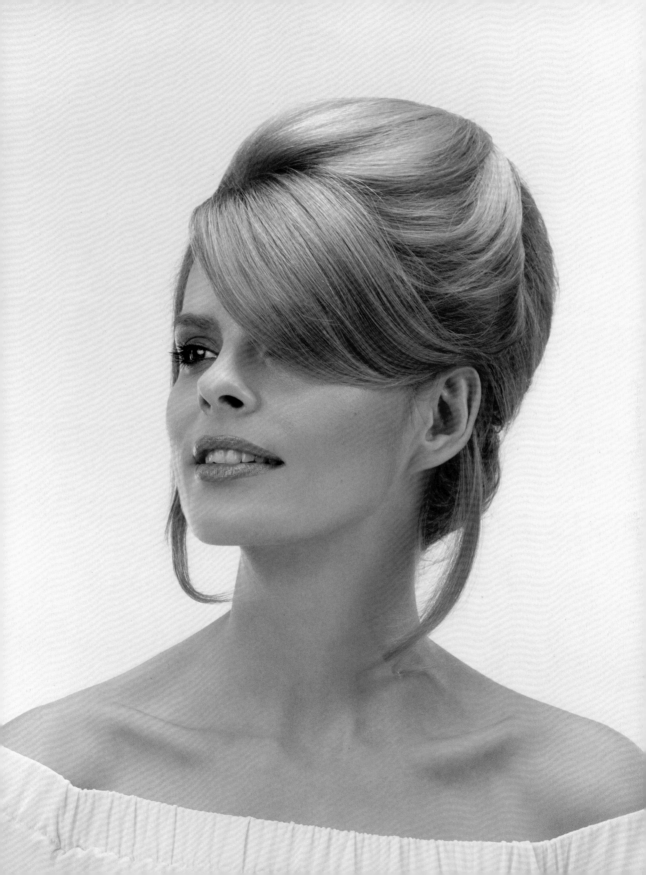

TWISTED HIGH CHIGNON

A cool updo for hair that's at least shoulder length, and either straight or wavy. Perfect for clubbing – or wear it as a statement daytime look, with boyfriend jeans and a shirt.

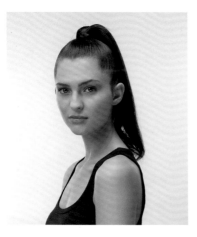

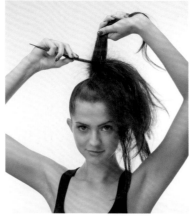

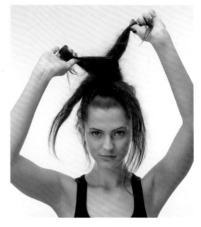

1. TIE BACK
Tilt your head forwards, brush your hair forwards and tie it into a ponytail at the highest point of your head, using a transparent hairband.

2. BACKCOMB
Divide the ponytail into several sections and backcomb them using a steel comb. You may want to add some mineral powder spray for better grip.

3. TWIST
Taking a backcombed section in each hand, lift and twist them around each other to form a long, tower-like chignon.

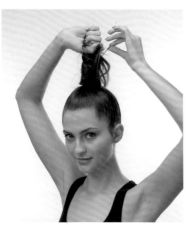

4. FIX
Pin the twisted sections securely in place with hairpins. Keep the look casual by allowing the ends to stick out. Fix with extra-strong hairspray for better hold and extreme shine.

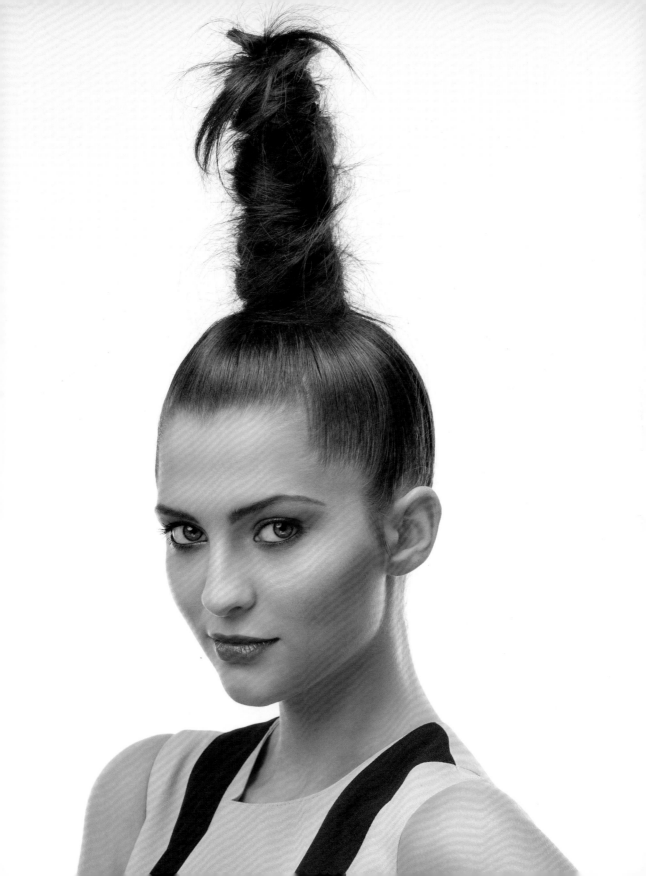

THE GRACE KELLY

That timeless favourite, the French roll, gets an unusual twist here, with a centre parting and long fringe section. The result is a glamorous yet casual updo that will make you feel like a movie star for a big night out.

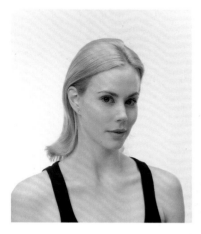

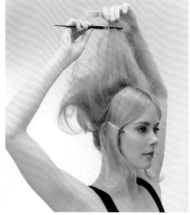

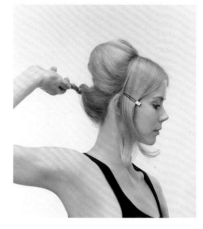

1. PREPARE
For this style, your hair should be at least shoulder length. Make a precise centre parting and brush the rest of your hair completely smooth.

2. BACKCOMB
Separate two thick side sections and clip them just above your ears. Backcomb the hair on the back and top of your head, adding some structure spray for better hold.

3. TWIST
Bring together the lower back section, tie it in the middle with a hairband, then twist and pin it into a mini French roll below the beehive section.

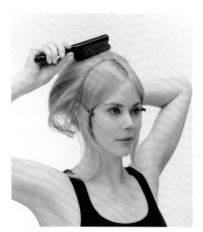

4. BRUSH
Brush the surface of the backcombed hair smooth, bringing it towards the back of your head. Turn the top section under and pin it in place, leaving lots of volume.

5. FIX
Backcomb the side sections thoroughly, then gently brush them out, sweep them back and pin at the back as invisibly as possible. Fix with hairspray.

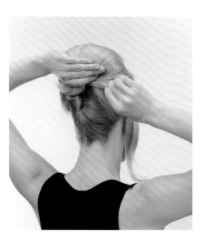

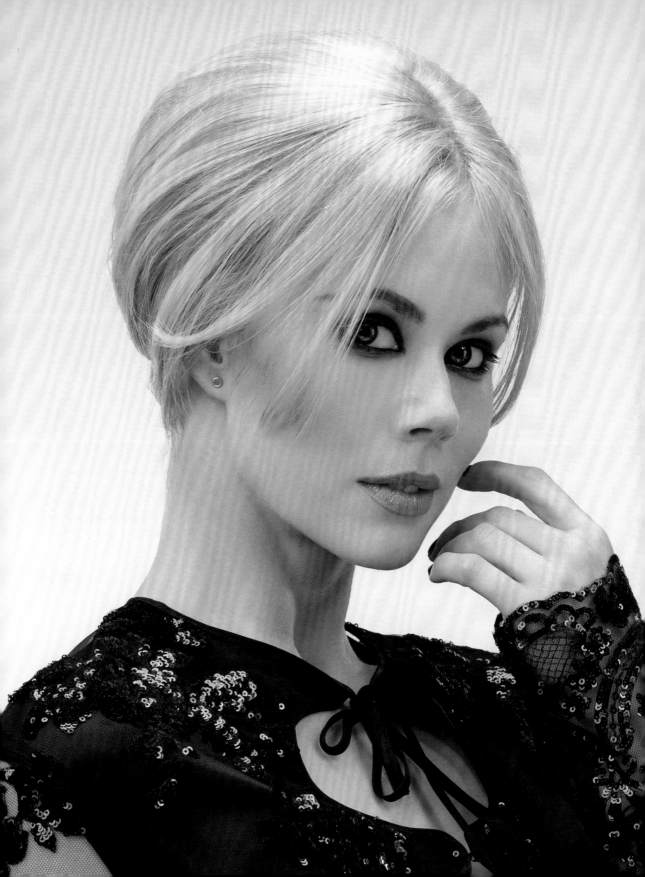

TWISTED UPDO

You'll get the hang of these twists in no time. They will give you an unusual chignon with maximum volume. This works best if your hair is thick and longer than shoulder length.

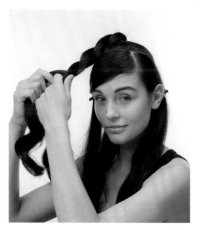

1. ROPE TWIST
Make a low side parting, and a horizontal parting a few centimetres above your ears. Make a ponytail from a thick strand from the top of your head, divide, rope twist and tie off.

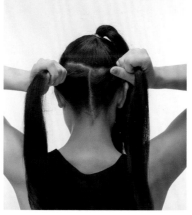

2. TWIST
Above the ear opposite the side parting, separate and clip back a thick strand. Divide the rest of the hair at the back into two thick strands and twist them.

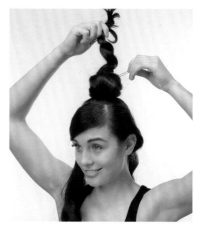

3. PIN
Pin the rope-twist ponytail into a loose bun with hairpins. If your hair is very thick and straight, add some structure spray for more grip.

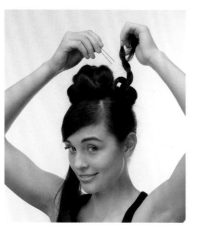

4. FIX
Pin up the two twisted sections in the same way, next to the bun. Unclip the fringe section, sweep it to one side and twist it inwards.

5. PLACE
Place the ends of the fringe section over the bun and pin them there with hairpins. Fix the whole thing in place and give it shine with strong hairspray.

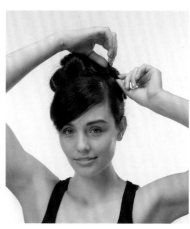

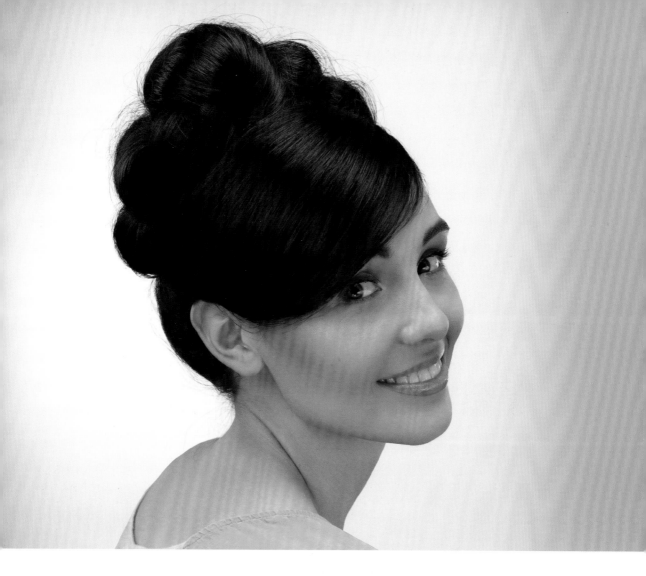

This piled updo creates interest at the back and a lovely profile, while the low fringe section flatters your face.

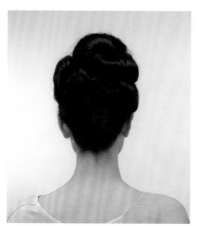

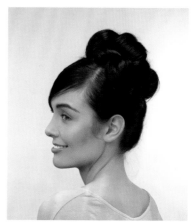

1 CUT – 4 LOOKS
LOOKS FOR LONG HAIR

It's a problem many women will be familiar with: you manage to grow your hair lovely and long, and then practical reasons (and a lack of ideas) make you hide it away in a simple ponytail day after day. These great ideas for day-to-day styling will let you do so much more.

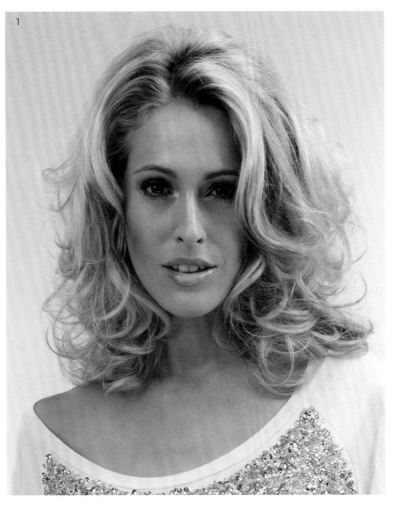

1. WILD
Want big hair, but with a casual look? No problem. Work a blob of styling mousse into your roots, dry your hair away from your head, and finally blow-dry using a round brush to give yourself lots of volume on top. Starting at ear level, wrap your hair around medium-sized curling tongs. Clip the curls up to let them cool as you go, until you've curled all your hair. Carefully remove the clips. Don't brush the curls out: just shape them with a little styling creme. Fix with lots of hairspray.

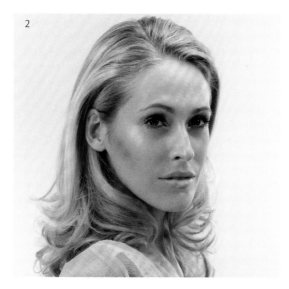

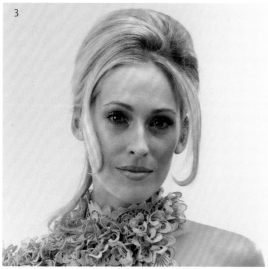

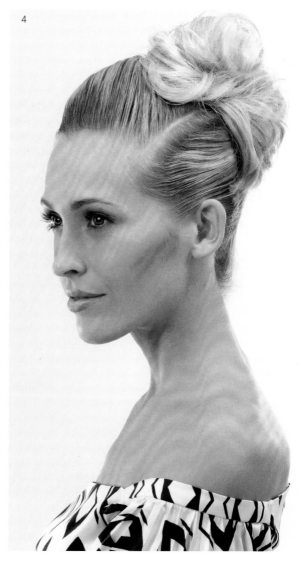

2. NATURAL

With the top section styled close to the head, and a light wave at the ends, this style has all you need for a very casual look. Blow-dry towel-dried hair straight using a paddle brush, then blow-dry the lower part of your hair with a mid-sized round brush to give the ends some movement. Smooth the side sections down with a little styling creme.

3. GLAMOROUS

The perfect look for a big occasion: a French roll with tons of volume, combined with soft strands falling over your face. Spray your hair with structure spray and backcomb it thoroughly with a steel comb. Brush it backwards and pin it into a loose French roll. Tease out a few thick strands at the front, sides and back.

4. STYLISH

A gorgeous look that's just made for a summer party. Make a very low side parting and brush your hair back from your face, adding lots of hairspray to your roots – it should look damp and shiny. Fasten it into a soft, asymmetrical bun, leaving the ends loose to drape around the bun. Hairspray will give you extra hold.

XXL CHIGNON

Want a voluminous updo that will make the most of your hair – even if it's fine? Work some hair magic with a clever backcombing technique, the right styling products, and a simple trick to finish.

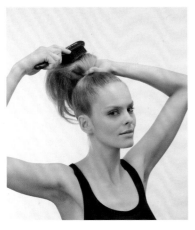

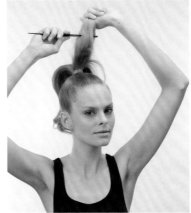

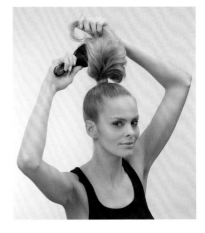

1. FASTEN
This style works for hair that is shoulder length or longer. Brush it into a high ponytail and fasten it with a transparent hairband.

2. BACKCOMB
Divide your ponytail into several sections and backcomb them one at a time with a steel comb. If your hair is very soft, use structure spray for added grip.

3. SMOOTH
Smooth the bushy backcombed sections back down with a brush. Retain the volume you've created by brushing only the surface hair.

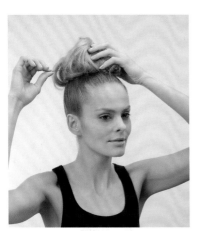

4. PIN
Pin your hair into a very loose chignon high on your head. The looser it is, the more volume you will have. Fix well with hairspray.

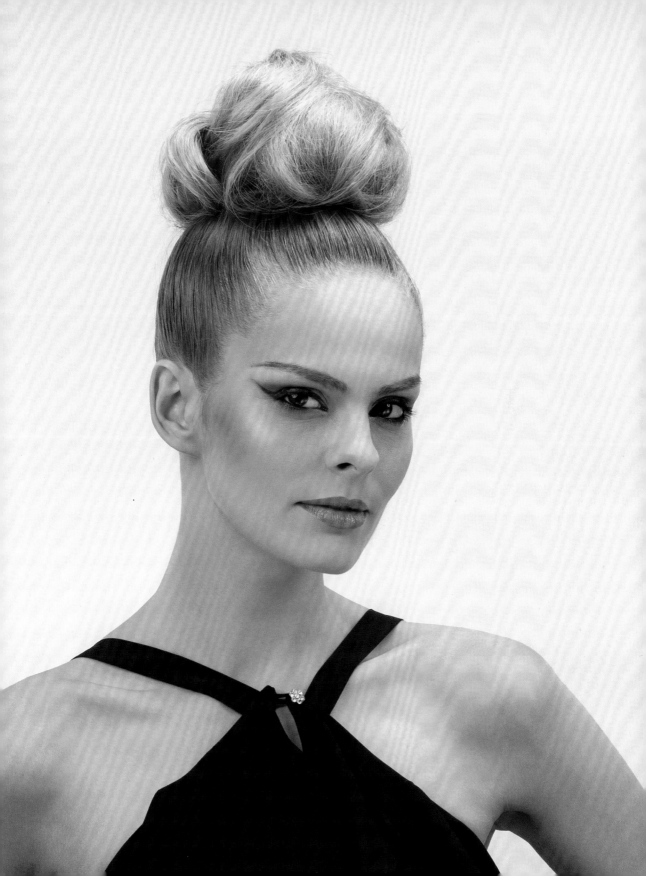

UPDO WITH A SPIRAL TWIST

Who says an updo always has to be on the back of your head? This look proves the opposite: an ornamental detail on your forehead will bring out beautiful eyes, flatter your face, and give you a sophisticated edge.

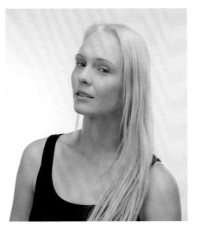

1. PREPARE
Hair should be well over shoulder length for this updo. Give the ends of your hair a little flick under with a hairdryer or curling tongs.

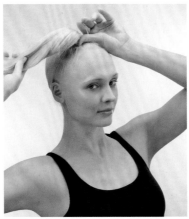

2. TIE
Brush all your hair into a ponytail at the front of your head, and tie it tightly with a transparent hairband.

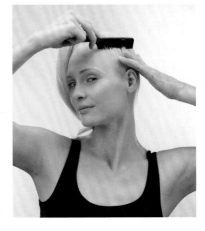

3. COMB SMOOTH
Spray some extra-hold hairspray onto the sides and smooth them with a comb. A damp, shiny look here just adds to the elegance.

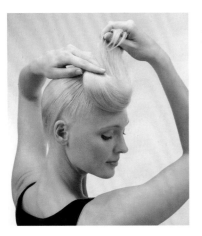

4. TWIST
Twist the ponytail into a spiral, making sure the hairband is completely hidden. Let the ends fall onto your forehead.

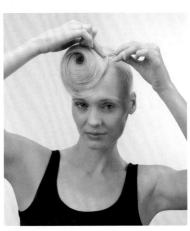

5. FIX
Use hairpins to fix the spiral in place as invisibly as possible. A generous amount of extra-strong hairspray will hold this extravagant style in place for a long time.

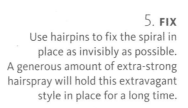

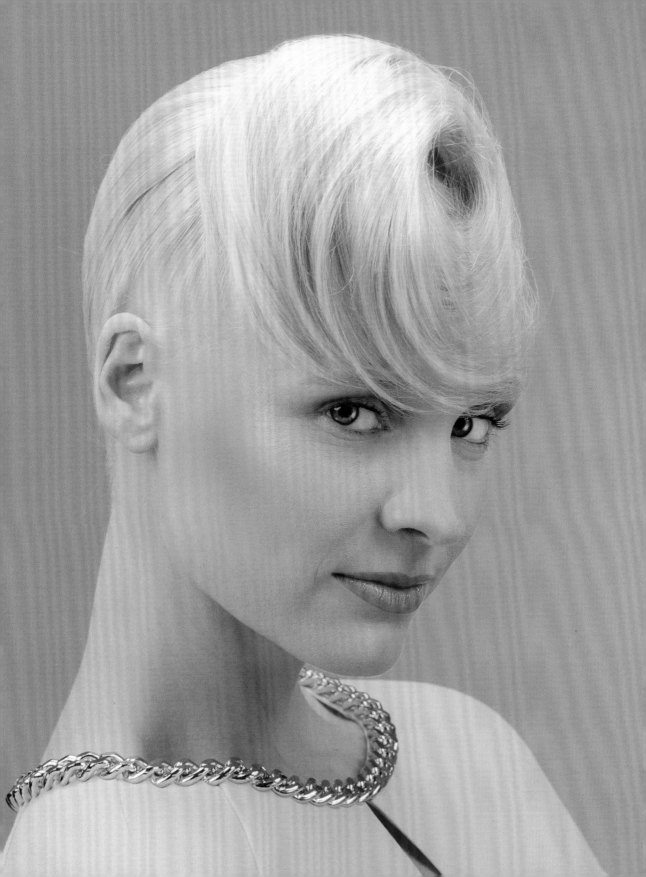

UPDO WITH A CLASSIC ROLL

Perfect for a job interview, elegant for a dinner date; this updo is a classic, but that doesn't make it old-fashioned. A little ornament at the back provides the finishing touch.

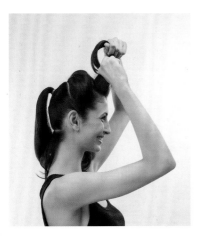

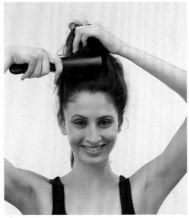

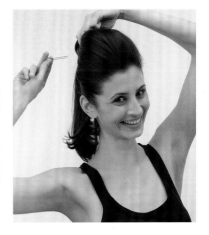

1. **DIVIDE**
Make a horizontal parting from ear to ear. Tie the back section into a high ponytail, leaving some hair at the nape of your neck loose.

2. **BACKCOMB**
Backcomb the front section thoroughly using a steel comb, and brush the surface smooth again with a styling brush.

3. **FIX**
Place the backcombed front section over the ponytail, twist it and pin invisibly with hairpins at the back of your head.

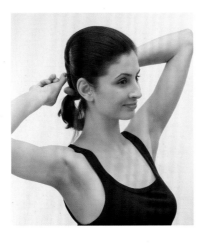

4. **WRAP**
Wrap the thin strands from the back of your neck around the twisted ponytail and pin them in place. Add a decorative clip as a finishing touch.

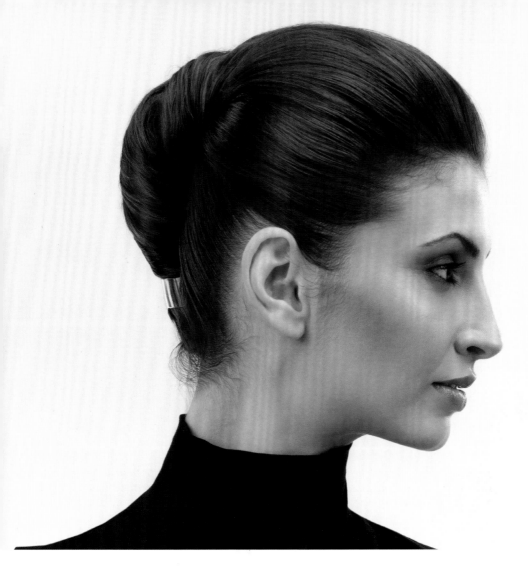

This updo highlights the forehead and the neck in a very elegant way.

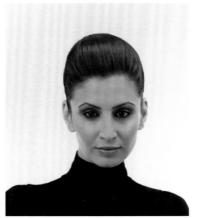

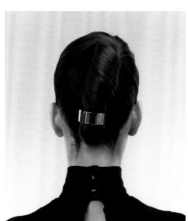

CASUAL FRENCH ROLL

Timeless beauty: the French roll is a classic look for any occasion.
Here is a very stylish version of the updo, which is perfect for work,
or for a date.

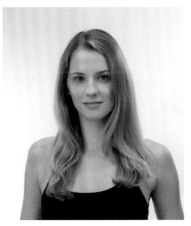

1. PREPARE
Your hair should be at least shoulder
length for this style. Soft waves or
curls are no problem, either. Brush
through, and work in some mineral
powder spray.

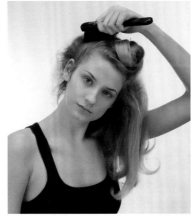

2. SEPARATE
Separate a rectangular section at the
front of your head, and clip it out of
the way. Brush the rest of your hair
over to one side.

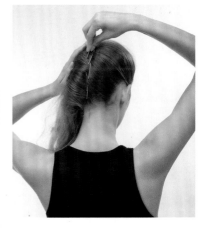

3. PIN
Spray some extra-hold hairspray onto
the loose hair, then hold it with one
hand as you pin it in place, with a
diagonal line of hairgrips down the
back of your head.

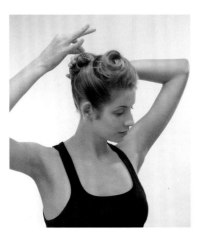

4. FIX
Twist this hair into a French roll in
the direction it has just come from.
Pin the roll in place securely and
invisibly with hairpins.

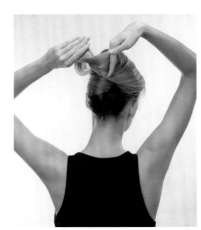

5. COVER
Unclip the front section and roll it
over the larger roll, in the opposite
direction. Pin it in place.

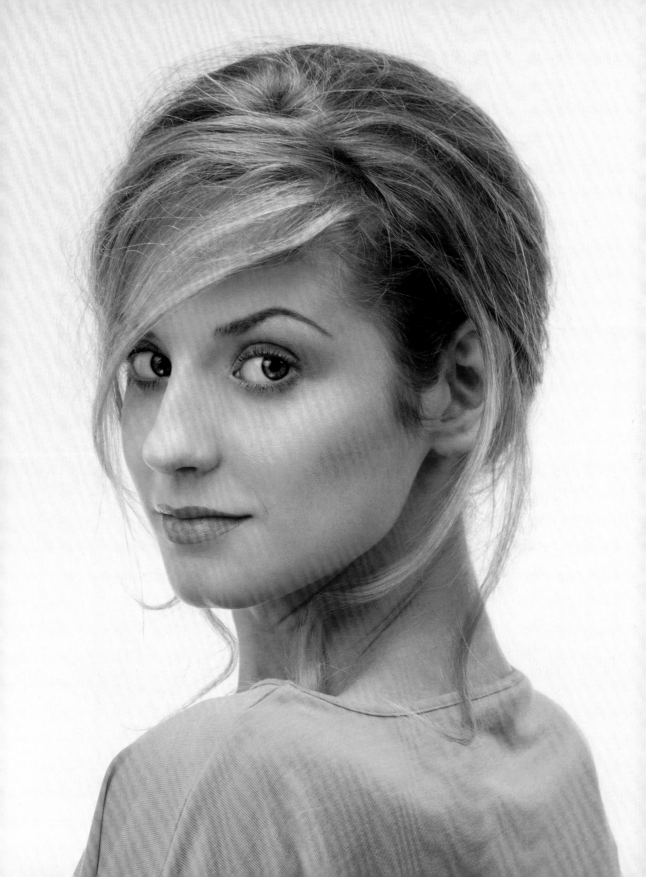

TWISTED CHIGNON

A bun is a bun is a... wait a minute... This is a chignon with a cute twist – quite literally! It looks very different to its simpler relatives. Twisting your hair gives it a unique structure after you've put it up.

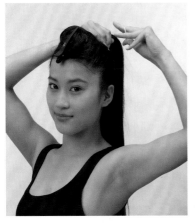

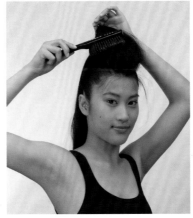

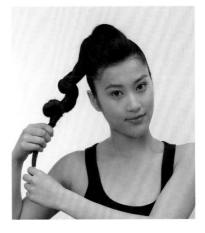

1. TIE
The longer and thicker your hair is, the better. Separate a section at the front of your head and clip it out of the way. Tie the rest of your hair into a high ponytail.

2. BACKCOMB
Backcomb the front section with a brush, then comb the surface smooth and bring it back over the ponytail. Use some structure spray for added grip.

3. TWIST
Take the ponytail in both hands, and twist it until it starts to coil up by itself.

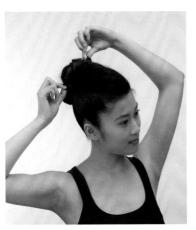

4. FIX
Make the twisted hair into a coil on top of your head, and pin it securely with hairpins. Add a lot of extra-strong hairspray for better hold.

5. BACK VIEW
Use a second mirror to check the back of your head: this is especially important with updos, to make sure your chignon is well-shaped and central.

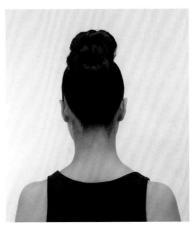

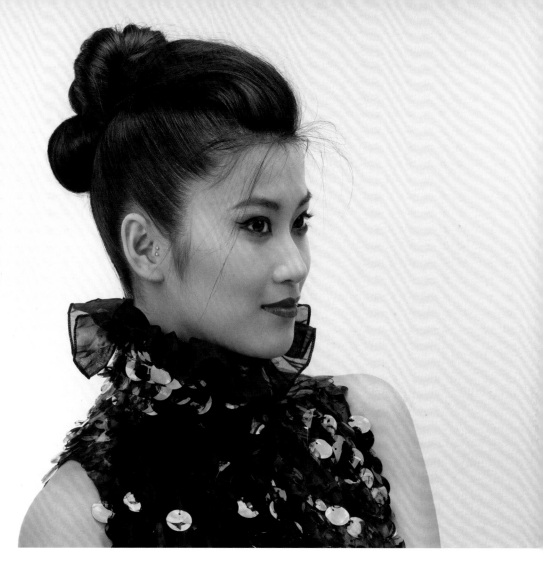

Très chic:
the twisted chignon
works as a daytime
or an evening look.

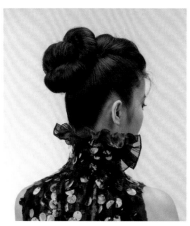

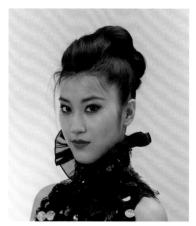

HIGH GLAMOUR ROLL

Sometimes you just have to think big. If you want to make a splash at a gala dinner, a ball, or your best friend's wedding, why not try this elegant, formal look.

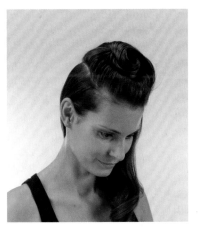

1. PREPARE
Use curling tongs to create voluminous curls, then separate the top front section of hair above your temples and clip it out of the way. Brush out the rest of your hair.

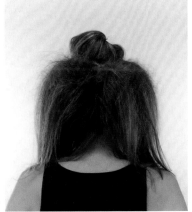

2. DIVIDE
Part the loose hair in the centre, all the way down to your neck. Add some structure spray to your roots on both sides, and backcomb them.

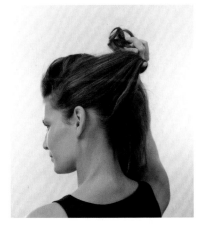

3. SWEEP
Smooth the surface of both sides with a brush, then sweep the left-hand section into a French roll in the middle and pin it in place invisibly with hairpins.

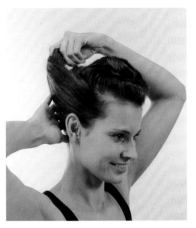

4. PIN
Do the same with the right side. Make sure the ends of your hair are hidden under the rolls on both sides.

5. DRAPE
Unclip the front section and backcomb it thoroughly. Brush the surface smooth, sweep back and roll under. Pin it above the double roll, leaving lots of volume on top.

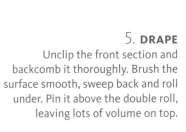

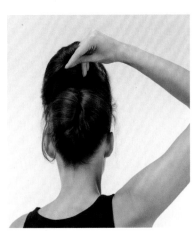

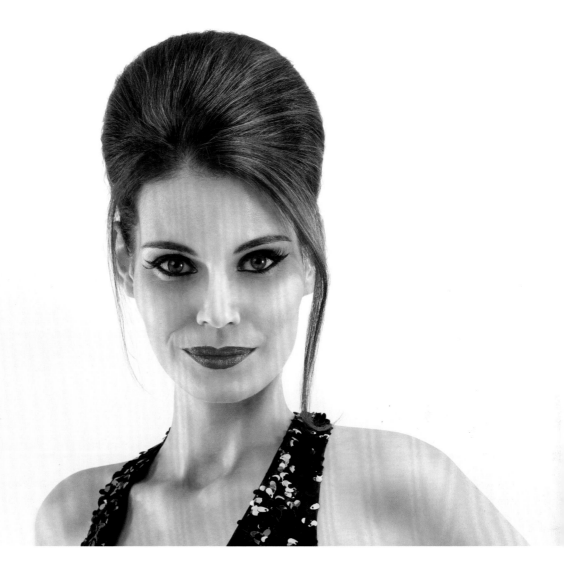

Asymmetrical: give this formal updo a cute touch with a loose strand over your forehead.

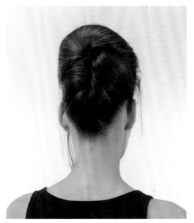

BASIC TECHNIQUES
HAIR ACCESSORIES

However good your style, great clips, classy grips, lacy flower bands or diamante pins will add a pretty touch to any look.

ACCESSORIES

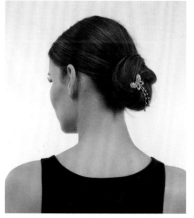

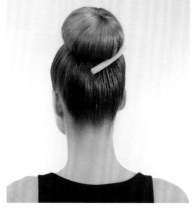

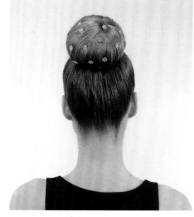

BUTTERFLY CLIP
A hairclip with a glittering butterfly gives the low, loose chignon a touch of romance. Tip: fix the chignon with hairspray before attaching the clip.

XXL CLIP
Placed diagonally and off-centre, this large, white clip acts like an exclamation mark after what is otherwise a classic, high chignon.

DIAMANTE PINS
Wear some sparkling flowers in your hair. Classy, luxurious, yet modest: lots of little diamante hairpins lend some glamour to this giant bun.

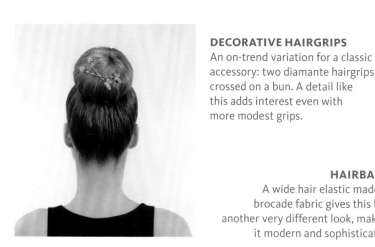

DECORATIVE HAIRGRIPS
An on-trend variation for a classic accessory: two diamante hairgrips crossed on a bun. A detail like this adds interest even with more modest grips.

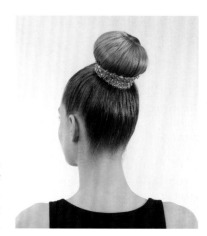

HAIRBAND
A wide hair elastic made of brocade fabric gives this bun another very different look, making it modern and sophisticated.

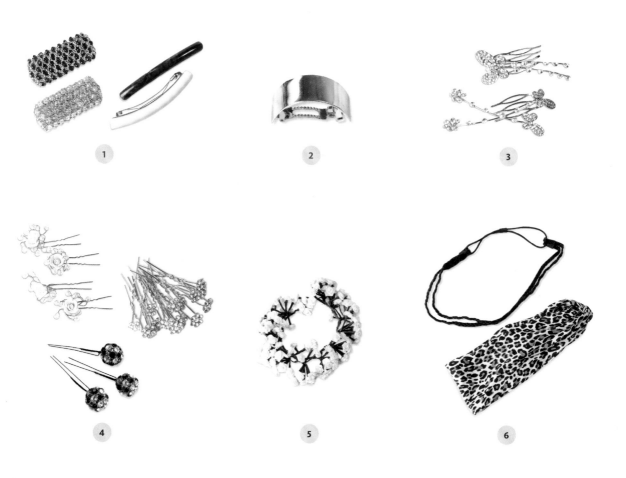

1. HAIR CLIPS
These come in different sizes and lengths, and are made of plastic or (for a classy look) horn.

2. PONYTAIL CLIP
A semi-circular metal clip is a great alternative to a classic hairband for a ponytail.

3. MINI COMBS
These can just be used as decoration, though wider ones can also hold an updo together.

4. HAIRPINS
Little bits of decoration like flowers or pearls can turn simple hairpins into a classy feature.

5. FLOWER ARRANGEMENT
Whether large or small, flowers make a really eye-catching feature. Don't use real flowers, as they dry out too quickly.

6. HAIRBANDS
Wide or narrow, patterned or plain – hairbands bring variety and can make a real difference to a hairstyle.

HIPPY CHIC WITH HEADBAND

Glastonbury; Coachella: it's impossible to imagine the world's biggest music festivals without the hippy look. Here, long, centre-parted hair is decorated with a soft, narrow band – girly and totally natural.

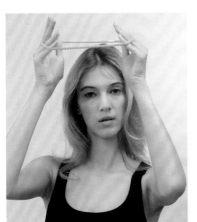

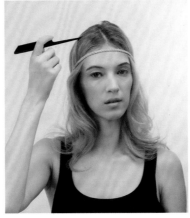

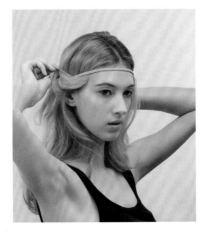

1. PUT ON
Give yourself a centre parting and brush your hair thoroughly. Hold the elastic headband from inside with both hands, and place it over your forehead.

2. LOOSEN UP
Push the end of a steel comb into the hair around the top of your head, and carefully loosen it up so that it doesn't lie too flat.

3. ROLL
Take a thin strand from above each ear, backcomb them lightly, and roll them back and inwards to form a soft wave. Pin them in place with hairpins.

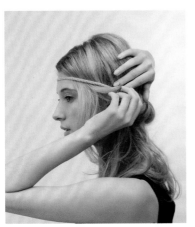

4. STYLE
Tease out a thin strand from your temples on each side and let them fall casually over your face. Spray with extra-strong hairspray.

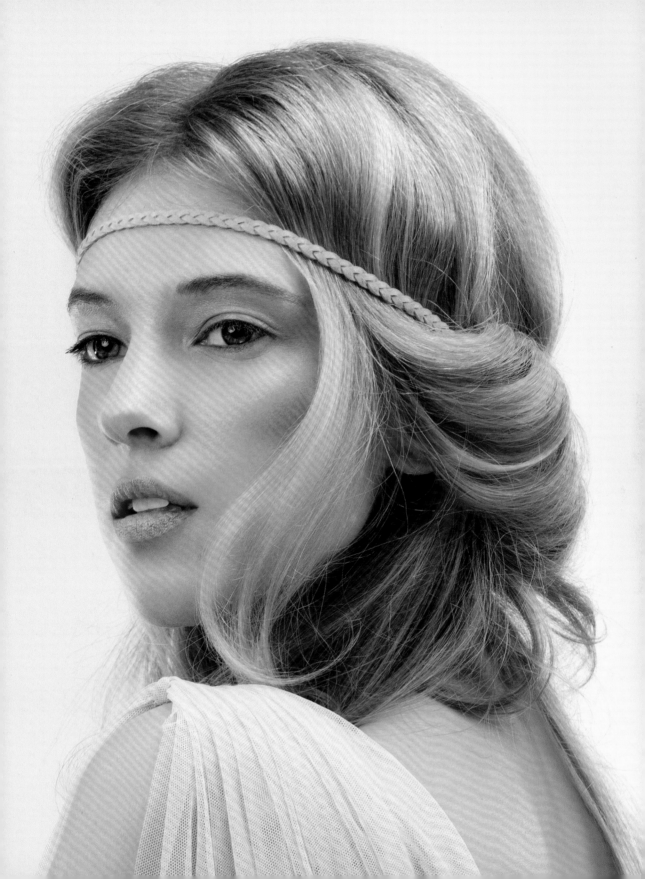

BEEHIVE WITH DIADEM

The It Girls of this world have shown us the way: the diadem is one of the hippest hair accessories going, making every hairstyle look like a crown. Here, it's used to decorate a classic beehive.

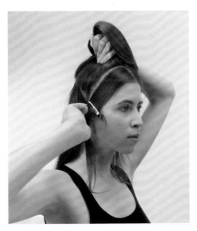

1. SEPARATE
Make a centre parting, separate a not-too-thin strand from above each ear and clip them in place. Make a horizontal parting across the back of your head from ear to ear.

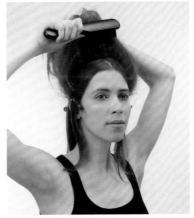

2. BACKCOMB
Use a brush to backcomb the hair on top of your head, one strand at a time. Add a little structure spray at intervals as you go.

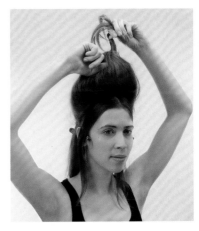

3. WRAP
Wrap the ends of the backcombed section loosely around two fingers, turn them under to form a tall beehive, and pin in place. This will form a pad for the side sections.

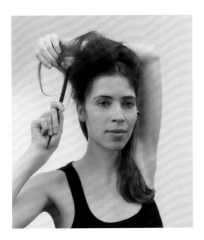

4. DEFINE
Unclip the sections above your ears and backcomb them with a steel comb. Brush the surface smooth and sweep them back along the sides of the beehive.

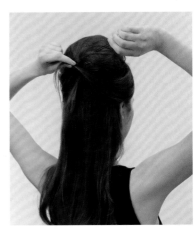

5. FIX
Pin the side sections securely high up on the back of your head, and fix with hairspray. Add the diadem as a crowning touch.

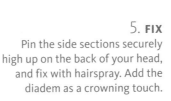

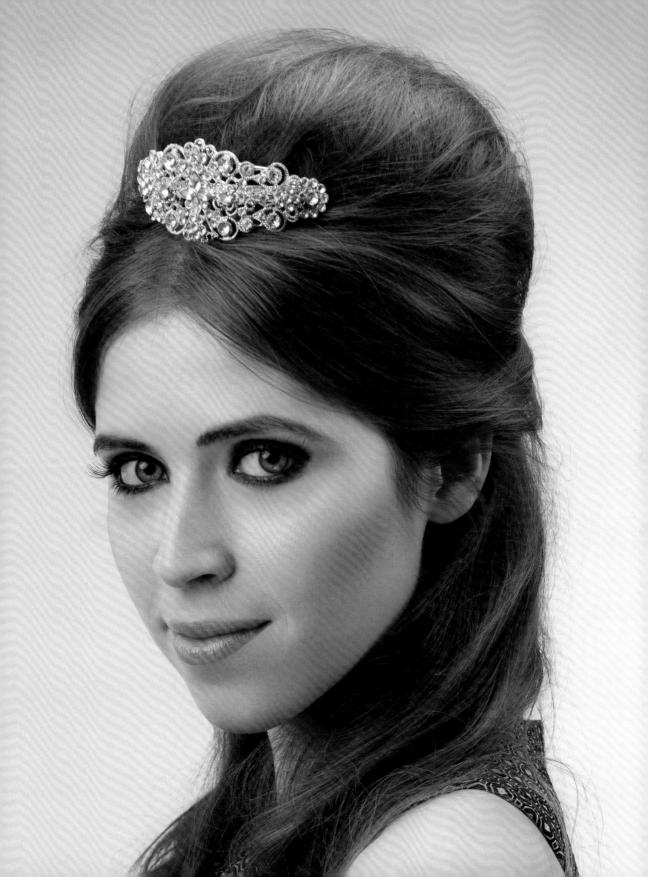

ROMANTIC ROLL WITH FLOWERS

A little bit hippy, a little bit ballerina. You can keep reinventing this dreamy updo by combining it with a surprising number of different outfits – from a floaty chiffon dress to hotpants and biker boots.

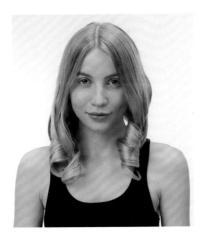

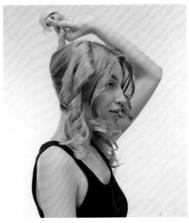

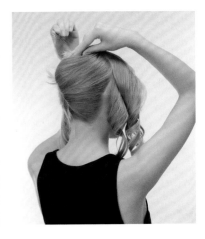

1. PREPARE
The romantic roll is ideal for hair that's at least shoulder length. Hair type isn't important – it works just as well with straight or wavy hair. Make a centre parting.

2. CURL
Divide each side section into four thick strands and curl each with large-barrelled curling tongs. Hold the curl in place, pull out the tongs, clip up and leave to cool.

3. ROLL
Bring the hair at the back of your head together and twist it around itself. Roll it into a high French roll, and pin invisibly with hairpins.

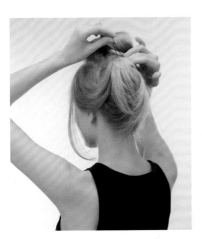

4. PIN
Brush out the curly side sections, backcomb them lightly and sweep them back. The French roll acts as a hair pad, giving you lots of volume at the back.

5. DECORATE
Turn the side sections inwards over the roll and pin them in place with hairpins. Decorate the updo with real or artificial flowers.

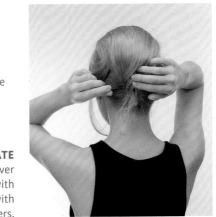

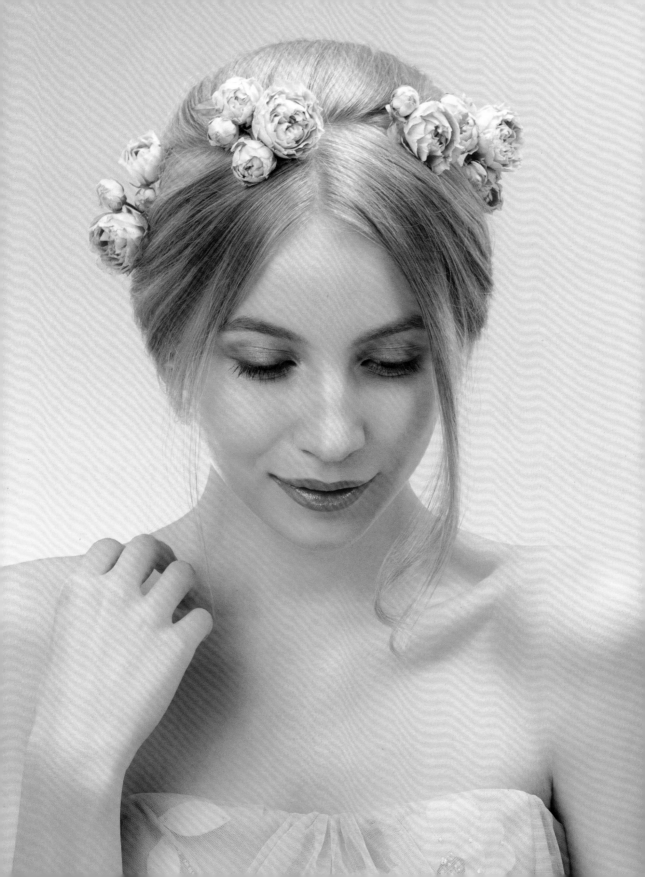

FLOWER POWER STYLE

Classic Flower Power with a modern twist: the flower headband sits low on your forehead, with a French-roll-type updo at the back.

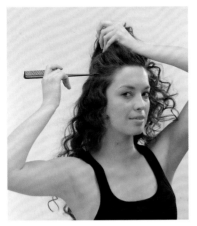

1. DIVIDE
Make a high horizontal parting from ear to ear with a steel comb, and bring the hair at the front together with your hands.

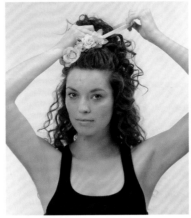

2. PUT ON
Put the flowered hairband over the hair you are holding, placing it on top of the back section, just above your ears.

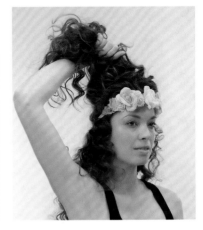

3. GATHER
Backcomb the top section lightly with a brush or steel comb, smooth the surface back down with your hands, and wrap into a loose French roll at the back of your head.

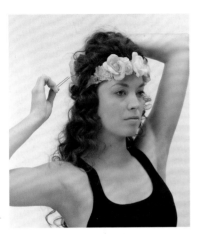

4. PIN
Use hairpins to pin the roll in place over the hairband, securely and invisibly. Make sure your hair isn't too tight against your head – this style needs some volume.

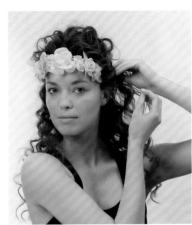

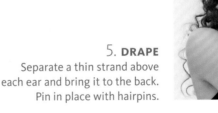

5. DRAPE
Separate a thin strand above each ear and bring it to the back. Pin in place with hairpins.

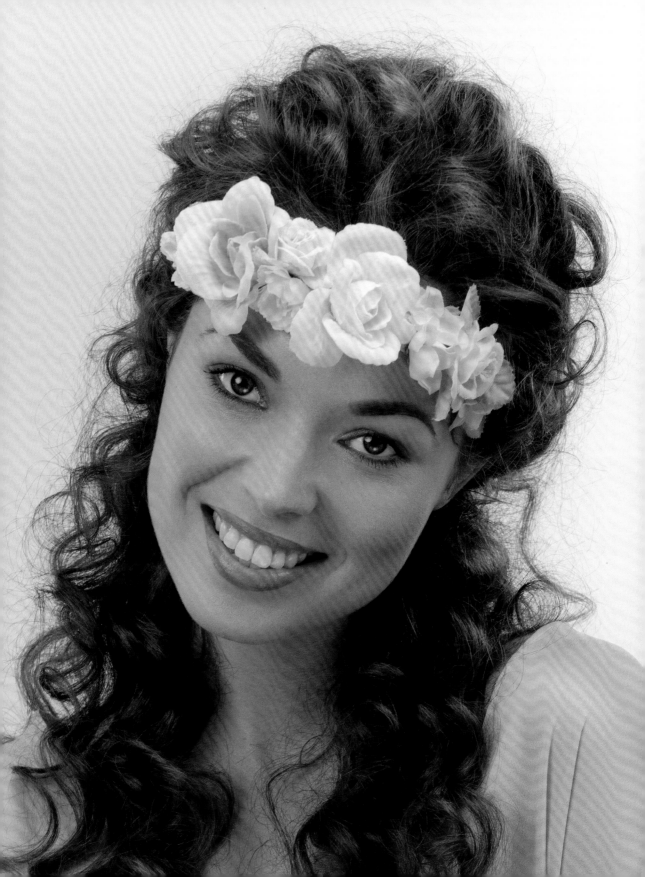

UPDO WITH HEADBAND

From the back, it's an elegant French roll; from the front, it's stylish and alternative: this extravagant updo with a decorative headband is classic and cool at the same time.

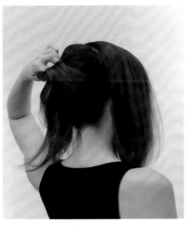

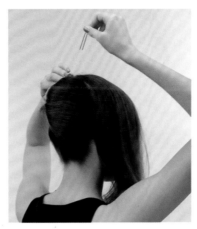

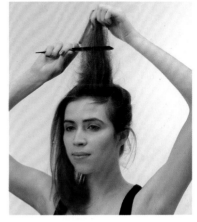

1. DIVIDE
Separate a section of your hair in front of your crown, down to your temples. Roll the rest of your hair, including the sides, into a French roll on the back of your head.

2. FIX
Pin the roll in place securely and invisibly with hairpins. It shouldn't look too neat – you're going for cool and casual!

3. BACKCOMB
Divide the top front section into strands and backcomb them thoroughly with a steel comb. Smooth the surface with a brush, and lay this section over the roll.

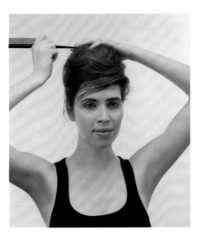

4. TEASE OUT
Tuck it under and pin in place. Carefully tease out some hair to give the style more body.

5. ADD YOUR BAND
Put both hands inside the headband, stretch it out as far as you can and carefully put it over the finished updo. Tease out some hair over your forehead.

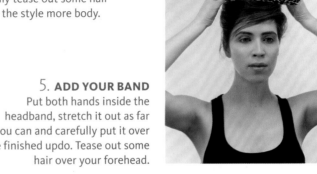

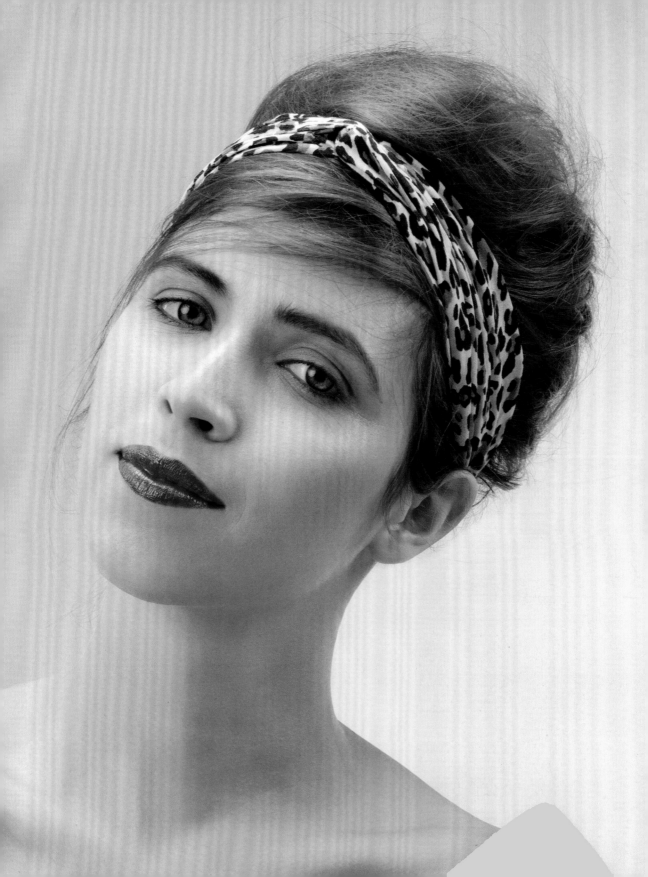

ALL PERFECTLY NORMAL: HAIR TYPES

Oily or dry scalps, brittle ends, greasy hair: there can be all kinds of causes for common hair problems. To some extent your hair type is genetic – all the rest is the result of hormones, environmental factors, and the right care regime.

GREASY HAIR

Greasy hair is caused by overactive oil glands, which can be activated by poor diet, hormonal changes, or stress. Greasy hair should be washed every day if necessary. It is a myth that frequent washing activates your oil glands. You can use a mild volumizing shampoo, as well as products for oily hair. You should always wash out conditioner very thoroughly, so that any residue doesn't weigh your hair down, and only apply it to the body and ends of your hair. Dry shampoos are a perfect in-between solution – they soak up oil like blotting paper. Styling products that keep your roots away from an oily scalp can help. These include setting mousse and hairspray – some of these contain a small amount of alcohol that has a slight de-greasing effect.

NORMAL HAIR

Is your hair silky to the touch, gleaming, and free from split ends? Congratulations on being one of the lucky few! To make sure your hair stays that way, choose the gentlest shampoo formula you can. And even uncomplicated hair will benefit from a conditioner and an occasional hair masque. If you use heat tools like hairdryers, straighteners, or curling tongs a lot, you should always apply a heat protection product. Overly frequent chemical shaping (e.g. perms or chemical straightening) can take its toll even on normal hair.

STRESSED HAIR

Hair is actually pretty easy going, and will put up with a lot: washing, blow-drying, colouring, straightening, perming, styling. But heap up all these little attacks, and it can start to get overwhelmed. The scales of the cuticle or outer layer, which normally lie flat like a closed pine cone, open out, making your hair rough and brittle. In the worst case scenario, your hair can end up looking like candy floss: dull and with no elasticity. Then it needs a rescue package, starting with shampoo. Massage the shampoo gently into your scalp and roots with your fingertips, not into the body and ends of your hair. You really must use a conditioner after washing, and very fine hair will benefit from a light leave-in product. Modern silicone formulas bind frizz and split ends together, and leave your hair looking much healthier. A touch of hair oil on the ends can also work wonders, and a weekly hair masque is a must.

COLOURED HAIR

To keep your hair looking beautiful for as long as possible after colouring, you should use a care range designed for coloured hair. It will give your hair the care it needs, and protect the colour from fading too quickly. Important: in summer, dyed hair really needs colour protection with a UV filter, in the form of a spray to be used before spending any time outdoors.

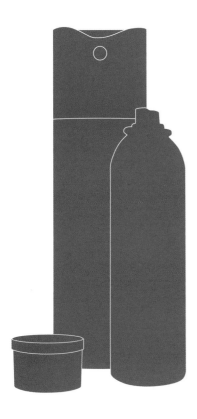

DRY/BRITTLE HAIR

Can be caused by stressful treatments, or a problem with the growth of your hair brought on by a lack of biotin. This vital substance is an important building block for keratin formation, and plays a crucial role in the healthy growth of skin, hair, and nails. Sometimes your scalp can also produce too little oil, making it feel itchy and tight. This can have a variety of causes, and means that the protective film of oil that covers the surface of healthy hair becomes too thin. This in turn leads to the hair cuticle becoming porous and rough, with nothing to prevent moisture from inside the hair evaporating. You can combat this with lipid replenishing oils, and silicones that seal in moisture.

A SENSITIVE PLANT: THE SCALP

A good hairdresser may well ask: "And how's your scalp doing?" There are plenty of reasons for looking after your scalp. Not least of all, its condition is crucial for the appearance and condition of your hair. Like the skin on your body, your scalp sends out an SOS from time to time. It can itch, burn, and feel tight. Sometimes it can even look red, and if this happens you'll often get oily or dry flakes as well. Like the rest of your skin, your scalp forms a protective layer against damaging influences from outside, and moisture loss from within. To put it simply, your scalp is a "wall" of lipids (fats) and dead skin cells. But influences like the climate, dry air from central heating, certain ingredients in care products, chemical procedures, and even stress, can lead to fewer lipids being produced. As a result, the protective layer becomes thin and permeable. Relief can come in the form of special calming shampoos for sensitive scalps, and an ultra-mild care routine. If these don't relieve your symptoms, you may want to consult a dermatologist. It's possible the chaos on your scalp is being caused by a fungal infection, which is quick and easy to treat with the right drugs and medicated shampoos.

DANDRUFF

Dandruff is caused by problems with the top layer of cells on the scalp. Possible triggers include over or under-functioning oil glands, problems with your inner organs, metabolic disorders, dry skin caused by unsuitable or aggressive care products, badly rinsed-out shampoo, dry air from central heating, stress, or other psychological issues. These make your skin lose its protective function, which allows microorganisms like bacteria or fungus to multiply on your scalp. The scalp reacts with increased production of dead skin cells, which then fall off as visible flakes. Dandruff is best treated every day with a mild anti-dandruff shampoo or a peeling preparation from your hairdresser, specifically formulated for over or under-functioning of the scalp. Both will calm the scalp and free it from residue by cosmetically removing flakes. A very mild cleansing routine is the key to preventing a build-up of dandruff, and getting rid of it permanently.

AHEAD BY A LENGTH: EXTENSIONS

Are you dreaming of truly big hair? Sadly, nature doesn't always give us the volume we want. But extensions can be the way forward: attached to your own hair in a flash, they'll create a real wow factor.

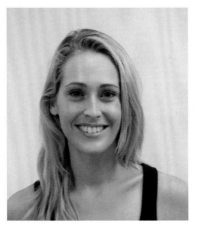

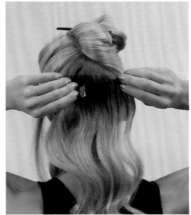

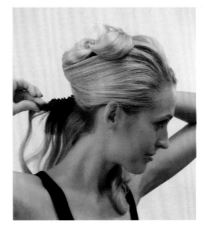

1. PREPARE
If your hair is layered and at least chin length, extensions will make it look longer and thicker. First of all, straighten or curl your hair, as you wish.

2. DIVIDE
Make the first dividing line across the back of your head, from ear to ear. Clip the hair above it out of the way and lay the clip-in hair piece along the line.

3. ATTACH
Work your way along the hair piece, attaching the mini clips to your roots. Make sure the extensions are attached securely to your own hair all the way along.

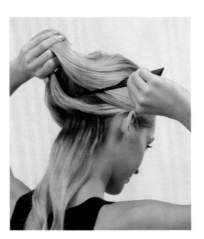

4. SEPARATE
Make the next dividing line 2–3cm (¾–1¼in) above the first. Clip the hair above it out of the way and attach another line of extensions, as above.

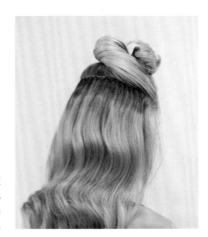

5. CHECK
Carry on until all your own hair is mixed in with the extensions. Brush through each section as you go.

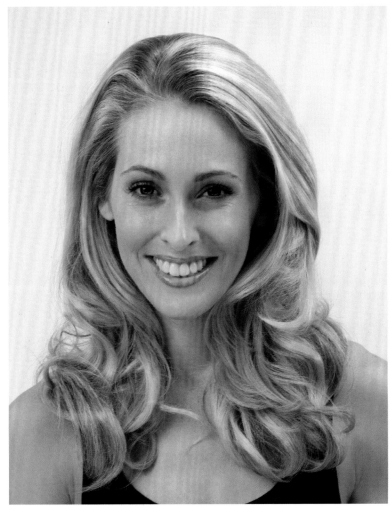

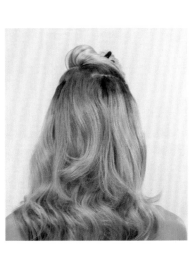

6. FINISH

Unclip the final, top section of your hair and lay it over the extensions. Be careful not to bring extensions too far round to the sides, or the clips will be visible.

Dream mane: the fake hair is impossible to distinguish from the real hair here, but it makes a huge difference.

FANTASTIC EFFECT

Think of clip extensions as hair you can wear for a special occasion, like a piece of jewellery or an evening dress. You can get reasonably priced artificial hair, or varying qualities of real hair. Artificial hair has a different structure from real hair. It also breaks more easily and can't usually be shaped with heat tools. Whatever kind of hair you choose, make sure the shade is as close as possible to your own hair colour. If you want to add permanent length or thickness, a hairdresser can bond extensions to your hair using a heat process – the best of which use natural-quality hair, coloured exactly to match your own. They can stay in for up to three months before the roots grow out enough to reveal the bond.

STRIKING THE RIGHT TONE: COLOURING YOUR HAIR

We've all seen celebrities whose hair is platinum blonde one day, a soft caramel shade the next, and brunette again the day after. A new hair colour can give you a whole new look. Here is what you need to know about the visual effects of hair colours, and using colour products.

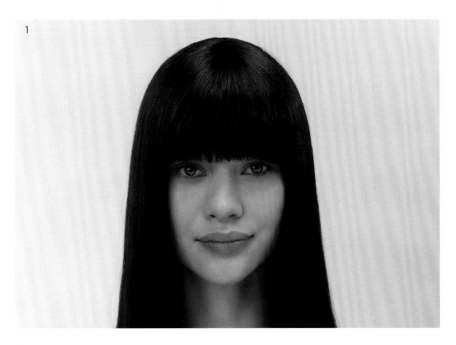

1. FROM CARAMEL TO HAZELNUT: BROWN

Brown is the new blonde - the colour is becoming more and more popular. The shade of brown that suits you is partly dependent on your skin tone and eye colour. If you have a rosy complexion with green or grey eyes, neutral browns with no red elements might be the best choice for you. Women with golden or olive skin and dark eyes are particularly suited to strong, dark chocolate shades. For a very light, even complexion, a shade of brown with a little red in it, like chestnut, can look very attractive. And blondes who dare to go brunette once in a while can try combining lighter shades, like golden brown, with gentle honey-blonde highlights.

TRY OUT A NEW COLOUR

Changing your hair colour completely can be a big step and you might want to make sure you will be happy about the result. If you're thinking about a complete change of colour, but don't know if it will suit you, there are websites where you can test the effect of the colour you want before you take you the plunge, by uploading a photo of yourself. Another option is to go to a specialist shop and try out a wig in that colour, if possible with a similar style to your own hair.

2

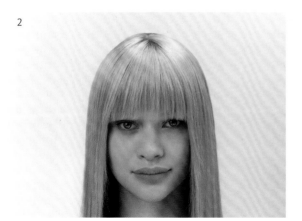

3

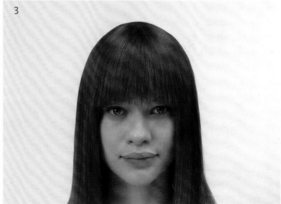

2. FROM PLATINUM TO HONEY: BLONDE

Natural blonde is a rare hair colour. These days, only one in every 15 blondes is "real". No matter: you can always give nature a little helping hand. Blonde has many facets. Ash blonde shades work best with a light tan, and look good cut into a geometric style such as a bob. But be careful if you have light, beige skin, as the lack of contrast with your hair colour can make ash blonde quite ageing. Golden blonde is a great summer colour, and looks good with a warm, bronzed complexion. It can be combined with highlights in warm or cool tones. Red-blonde shades suit warm skin tones, but can also look great with a very light, porcelain complexion.

3. FROM COPPER TO MAHOGANY: RED

Red is more than a hair colour: it's a statement. Only a small number of people have naturally red hair (though for Scottish people, the figure is 14 per cent, and 10 per cent for Irish people). Many more add an exclamation mark to their style by colouring their hair in shades of red. But all reds are not equal, and not every shade suits every skin type. Warm, yellowy, copper tones suit fair-skinned women with freckles – just as nature intended. Blueish-red shades suit very pale, even skin. As a general rule, be careful with red hair if your skin can get very flushed, or tends towards enlarged thread veins. Any additional red is not advisable.

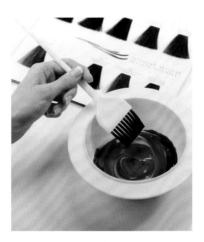

MIXING DYES

Mix the two components of the dye – usually a colour cream or gel and a liquid developer – in a plastic or glass bowl. Never use metal. Stir the two parts together with a plastic colour brush until they form an emulsion. Always use straight away.

FIND YOUR COLOUR

Most women guess their own hair colour to be much darker than it actually is, and therefore go for a dark dye. But what hairdressers would call a dark blonde, for example, looks like light brown to many amateurs. Tip: you will find sample strands with the hair dyes in specialist shops. Hold them up against your own hair in front of a mirror.

ALL COLOURS ARE NOT EQUAL

Permanent colours are distinguished by the fact that you have to mix two components together before use. During the colouring process, a pigment exchange takes place. First, the natural pigment in the hair is depleted; then comes a second step in which the new, artificial pigment is absorbed. Ammonia or an alkali alternative open up the outer layer of the hair follicle. Semi-permanent colour, colour mousse and colour conditioner, on the other hand, just deposit colour temporarily on the outside of the hair. This means the colour washes out gradually.

THE NUMBERS GAME

Hair dye packaging often has a number as well as the name of the colour. The first number in the colour code (from 1 to 10, though some manufacturers go up to 12) stands for the depth of colour. This relates to natural colours, from black (1) to a very light blonde at the top of the scale. The second number gives you the hair colour's tone. Zero stands for a natural tone, then ash (1), gold (2), copper (3), mahogany (4), red (5), and violet (6).

GENTLY DOES IT

Avoid changing your hair colour all the time. Celebrities who are red one day and blonde the next are often wearing wigs or hairpieces. And colour change belongs firmly in the hands of a professional, who will be an expert judge of the starting shade and will be able to choose a suitable, individually tailored colour.

PLANNING IS EVERYTHING

If you are colouring at home, read the instructions on your product carefully before you start. Then lay out everything you need, including a timer. Wear something to protect your clothes, like an old T-shirt, and use the protective gloves provided.

NO STRESS

Even if modern formulas and nourishing ingredients have made the colouring process very mild, don't put your hair through too much stress at once. There should always be at least a two-week gap between colouring and any chemical treatment (perming/chemical straightening).

BLONDE MOMENTS

You really need expert knowledge when colouring from dark to light. Is your hair already coloured? How light or dark is the natural shade? The darker it is, the more complex the lightening process will be. From a number 4 (mid-brown) and up, hair is pre-dyed blonde and then treated with a strong lightening hair colour. If hair is even darker, it will need to be bleached more and then coloured with the desired shade, perhaps using a semi-permanent colour. The bigger the colour gap, the quicker and more clearly you will start to see dark roots coming through.

STRIPY HAIR

The more continuously you use a hair colour, the more lovely and even it will become. Make sure you keep everything the same: that goes for the mix proportions, as well as the leave-on time and the intervals at which you dye your hair. This should be no more or less than four weeks. The older the uncoloured hair is, the more strongly it will keratinize, and your colour may not look as even. This goes for blonde shades in particular.

STRANDS

Be careful when using dyes containing bleach at home. Foils in particular are extremely tricky! The biggest danger is that the bleach or dye will leak out of the foil and colour your roots. Once the chemicals are covered up, they also work much more quickly and intensively, so you have to be even more precise about the leave-on time. With each foil, the time starts as soon as you add bleach or colour.

HIDE YOUR ROOTS

Lightening sprays only have a concealing effect if your own natural shade is already very light. The darker your roots, the less sense it makes to use them. They can lead to yellowy tones in your hair. Another problem is that the oxidation process is not stopped after a leave-in time, as it is with a bleaching process. Once they have been sprayed on, lightening sprays carry on working until you wash you hair. This "creeping oxidation" can do lasting damage to your hair and its sensitive roots.

SHINING LIGHTS

Bleaching is a stressful process for hair – especially if you want to transform a relatively dark starting colour into really light locks. The process is also quite tricky: if you wash the colour mixture out too soon, your hair can end up looking yellow or orange. Leave it in too long or use too high a concentration of hydrogen peroxide, and your hair can take on a rubbery quality, or even break. The best thing is to leave the treatment to a hairdresser. He will know exactly how long blonde dye needs to be left in, and will keep hair damage to a minimum.

SOS TIPS

Damage, drama, and disaster: there are days when everything just goes wrong. Unfortunately, that also goes for hair care and styling. But it won't matter as long as you know the most effective ways to rescue your hairstyle.

TOO MUCH WAX

It can happen all too quickly: dip a bit too deep into the wax pot, and suddenly your hair looks greasy. There's only one remedy: wash it – or comb it back into a shiny, sleek-look ponytail, if your hair is long enough. For short hair, reaching for the shampoo is often the quicker and simpler solution.

HAIR COLOUR TOO DARK

If you colour your hair at home, there's always a risk you'll go for the wrong shade. If your hair colour comes out too dark, the following trick will help: wash your hair twice with an anti-dandruff or peeling shampoo, then apply a hair masque and leave it in for at least an hour. The shampoo opens the hair cuticle a little, while the masque will remove some of the pigment from your hair, and nourish it at the same time.

FLAT ROOTS

Yesterday you spent hours styling your hair, and this morning it's pressed flat against your head. Try perking it up with the help of a little volumizing powder, massaged into the roots with small circular motions. If that doesn't work, massage some styling mousse into the roots and blow-dry your hair with a paddle brush against the direction of growth. It will soon stand up again.

OIL SLICK

If there's no time to wash your hair, but it looks greasy and badly needs refreshing, just spray on a little dry shampoo, massage it in for a minute and then brush it out thoroughly.

KINKY HAIR

Hair clips and bands often leave impressions and kinks behind, especially in freshly washed hair. There are special spiral-shaped hairbands that don't leave these dents. Otherwise, you can try this blow-dry trick: moisten the area with water, a little mousse or styling spray, and blow-dry over a large round brush.

FLY-AWAY HAIR

In winter, when you come into a much warmer room out of the cold, and especially if you are wearing a woolly hat, your hair can suddenly develop an electric charge and become fly-away. First tip: never brush or comb your hair straight away, it will only make you look more like Einstein. Second tip: spray some water into the air above your head with a plant mist spray, and carefully run your hands over your hair. That should bring it back down to earth.

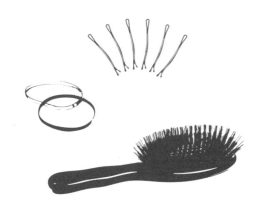

FRIZZY HAIR

You've just styled your hair perfectly – then you go out into damp air, and suddenly little hairs are sticking up everywhere. Experts call it frizz, and there is a remedy for it: rub a pin-head-sized amount of hair wax between warm hands, and then run them over your hair – or use an anti-frizz spray.

A SHADE TOO RED

An inadvertent red tinge after colouring your hair can be gorgeous, but it can also make you look pale. If necessary, cover it with a permanent or semi-permanent dye in an ashy or neutral shade to hide the red pigment.

UNTAMEABLE CROWN

Your crown can be a real pain when you're styling your hair. Here is how to temporarily tame it: spray a little styling spray onto its roots, smooth the hair down with a hairdryer and paddle brush, and fix with lots of strong hairspray. Never style against your crown: it can make your hair break! It's better to find a style where your crown can be integrated naturally and elegantly.

ORANGE ON BLONDE

If you don't leave hair dye on for long enough when you're going blonde, the result is often an ugly orange tinge. If this happens, you really need to seek professional help. A hairdresser can usually save your hair colour without too much stress.

BURNED SCALP

This can happen before you know it, especially if your hair is blonde and/or thin: after a long day at the beach, or in the evening on a summer city break, your parting or even your whole head will look sunburnt. SOS remedy: rub some aloe vera gel into your scalp. This will have a lovely cooling effect, reduce the inflammation, and is not oily. Even better: avoid the situation in the first place by wearing a hat during the day.

POST-POOL GREEN HAIR

Does your hair suddenly develop a green sheen after a dip in the pool? Dyed blonde hair doesn't like chlorine, and can have a chemical reaction to it. Rinsing your hair with two tablets of acetyl salicylic acid in a litre of still mineral water should help. Avoid green hair by wearing a swimming cap, even if it doesn't look very chic.

NO HAIRDRYER

You're travelling, and there's no hairdryer in the hotel room. Don't subject your hair to a rough rub with a towel: let it air dry. Pin up longer hair into a secure knot on the back of your head while it dries. Keep scrunching curls and waves together during the day.

CAMOUFLAGE FOR YOUR ROOTS
If you dye your hair, you will usually start to see the roots after four weeks. And if you don't have time to top up your colour, you can always use eyebrow mascara, which comes in various colours. Just sweep the brush over the roots, and in mid-blonde to black hair the coloured gel will hide any grey or dark regrowth until your next wash.

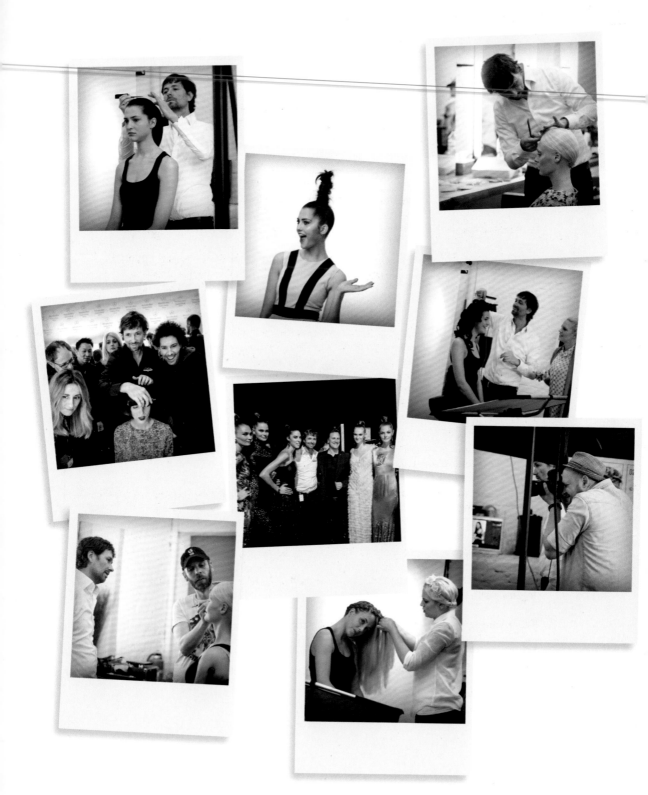

ACKNOWLEDGMENTS

Thanks to Gerhard Roll, who brought me to the Harder hairdressing school in Duisberg, and to my teachers Hans Becks, Dirk Glass and Michael Prinz, who taught me the fundamentals of this profession. Thanks to my friend Ralf Lutter, who took my first photos, and to Bernd Michalke, Günter Backhaus, Horst Fett, and Kerstin Lehmann and Gabriele Legouez from L'Oréal, who supported and believed in me.

Thanks to Ekaterina Schmuhl for the perfect cast for this book.

A thousand thanks to Eugen Mai for his perspective, and for the wonderful pictures.

Many thanks to all the designers for the beautiful outfits: Blacky Dress, Dimitri, Elisabetta Franchi, Elisabetta Franchi Gold, Ella Singh, Ewa Herzog, Four Flavor, Guido Maria Kretschmer, Guido Maria Kretschmer ebay-Kollektion, H&M, Irene Luft, Mango, Marcel Ostertag, Matthias Ophoff, Pull&Bear, Sack's, Wolford, Zara, Zara W&B Collection.

Heartfelt thanks to all the models, who made themselves available for this book with good grace and total dedication. And not forgetting their agencies, who were kind enough to support this project: Agnieszka B., Aicha Hanna M./Procast, Amira Elisa S./Procast, Anna-Lea B., Anne L./Modelpool, Buki A./4Play, Carmelina C./Modelpool, Carolin S., Claudia B./Procast, Cora M./Procast, Dora/Procast, Fata H., Germaine Shakira M./Volta Models, Jennifer S./McFit-Models, Katarina P., Katharina D., Katrin B., Lena L./Procast, Linda B./Modelfabrik, Luzie G./Procast, Lynn G./Volta Models, Maria B./Modelfabrik, Maria S./Splendide, Michaela S./ Most Wanted Models, Mirela K., Nele H., Olga P./Procast, Paulina/4Play, Peo S./Procast, Rebecca K., Rixa Christina W./Procast, Sarah R./Procast, Sophie Luise S., Stephanie W., Sussan Z./Volta Models, Tu Anh L. T.

Thanks to my wonderful team at the salon, who inspire me and give me the freedom to make projects like this a reality.

Thanks to my on-set assistant, Nadine Brönner, to Michael Schmidt for the great make-up, to Nabil El-Rayan for the styling, and Silke Amthor for finding the right words.

To Monika Schlitzer at Dorling Kindersley – many thanks for your faith in my work, and for letting me do this book.

Thank you, my dear Sigi, for opening so many doors for me – you're the best.

Thank you to my wonderful parents: my skilled father and my talented mother, from whom I was able to learn what might just be the best job in the world.

For my son.

Thank you, Susann.

ANDRÉ MÄRTENS

With 100 years of family tradition behind him, native Berliner André Märtens found it easy to decide on a career: he started by training as a hairdresser in his parents' salon, and at the renowned Friseurfachschule Harder in Duisberg. He has been running his own salon in Berlin since 2000. He is not only a long-hair expert; his name stands for performance, quality, and delightfully simple, elegant shapes. His talent as a hair stylist and trend-setter means he is in demand among professionals and as an advisor for customers in the media – as the hair expert at Guido Maria Kretschmer's side, for example, on the TV show "Hotter than my daughter". André Märtens also works as a hair artist on fashion shows, adverts, video and film productions, musicals, theatre, competitions, presentations and professional training events. As an ambassador for L'Oréal Professionnel, André Märtens has spent many years styling celebrities for public appearances and top models for international fashion shows. André Märtens has been "Head of Hair" and the principal Créateur behind almost all the looks at the Mercedes-Benz Fashion Week Berlin for L'Oréal Professionnel. In his Berlin salon, André Märtens's customers include people from the world of politics and economics, and numerous celebrities. André Märtens has the eye of an international master, and a passion for hair.

ANDRÉ MÄRTENS
Lietzenburger Straße 83
10719 Berlin
Tel. +49 30 88709500
www.andremaertens.de

ANDRÉ MÄRTENS MANAGEMENT AND PR
BrandFaktor . Die Markenmacher . Sigrid Engelniederhammer
Georgenstraße 5 . 80799 München . Tel. +49 (0)89 3837715 12
www.brandfaktor.com

EUGEN MAI

Eugen Mai is a photographer based in Berlin. He is young, experienced, and places an emphasis on the aesthetic quality of his pictures. He is responsible for multi-media experiences in the areas of fashion, advertising, and film. As a photographer and an art director, his focus is on producing emotionally charged images, where naturalism and elegance go hand in hand. www.eugenmai.com

Penguin Random House

PHOTOGRAPHY Eugen Mai
ADDITIONAL PHOTOGRAPHY Edward Schmuhl, Thomas Rafalzyk
CASTING Ekaterina Schmuhl
HAIR André Märtens
HAIR ASSISTANT Nadine Brönner
MAKE-UP Michael Schmidt
STYLING Nabil El-Rayan
TEXT BY Silke Amthor
EDITOR Julia Niehaus
DESIGNER Diana Dörfl

DK GERMANY
PUBLISHING DIRECTOR Monika Schlitzer
PROJECT EDITOR Andrea Göppner, Katharina May
PRODUCTION DIRECTOR Dorothee Whittaker
PRODUCTION COORDINATOR Katharina Dürmeier
PRODUCER Sophie Schiela

DK UK
TRANSLATOR Ruth Martin
PROJECT EDITOR Anna-Selina Sander
MANAGING EDITOR Dawn Henderson
MANAGING ART EDITOR Christine Keilty
SENIOR JACKET CREATIVE Nicola Powling
JACKET DESIGN ASSISTANT Laura Buscemi
JACKET CO-ORDINATOR Francesca Young
SENIOR PRE-PRODUCTION PRODUCER Tony Phipps
PRODUCER Jen Scothern, Olivia Jeffries
DEPUTY ART DIRECTOR Maxine Pedliham
DESIGN DIRECTOR Phil Ormerod
PUBLISHER Peggy Vance

DK INDIA
ASSISTANT EDITOR Maithilee Bhuyan
DEPUTY MANAGING EDITOR Bushra Ahmed
MANAGING ART EDITOR Navidita Thapa
PRE-PRODUCTION MANAGER Sunil Sharma
SENIOR DTP DESIGNER Pushpak Tyagi
DTP DESIGNER Manish Chandra Upreti

First published in Great Britain in 2015 by
Dorling Kindersley Limited
80 Strand, London, WC2R 0RL

Copyright © 2015
Dorling Kindersley Limited
A Penguin Random House Company

2 4 6 8 10 9 7 5 3 1
001–284985–Sep/2015

A CIP catalogue record for this book
is available from the British Library.

ISBN: 978-0-2412-1608-8

Printed and bound in China

Discover more at www.dk.com

A WORLD OF IDEAS:
SEE ALL THERMAYBE WEE IS TO KNOW